AF598101

Neutrophils

Edited by Maitham Khajah

Published in London, United Kingdom

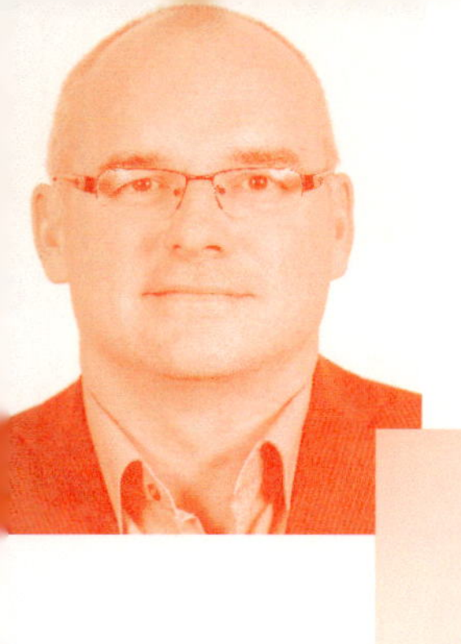
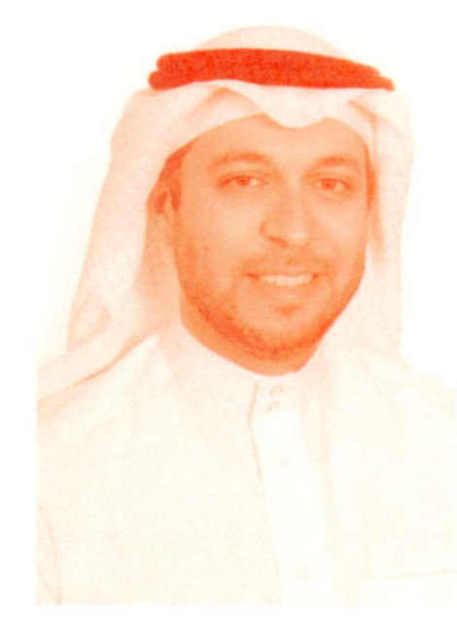
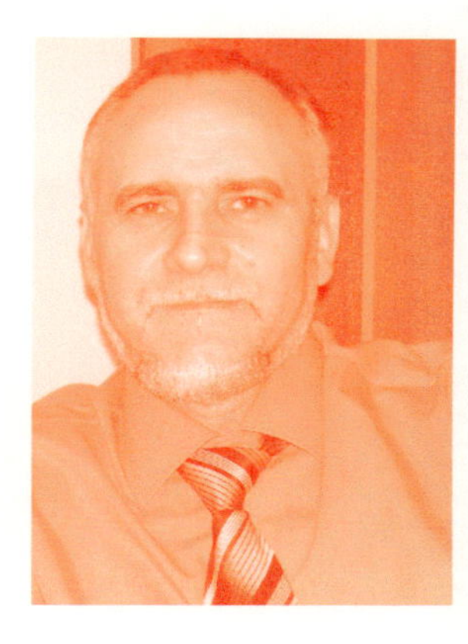
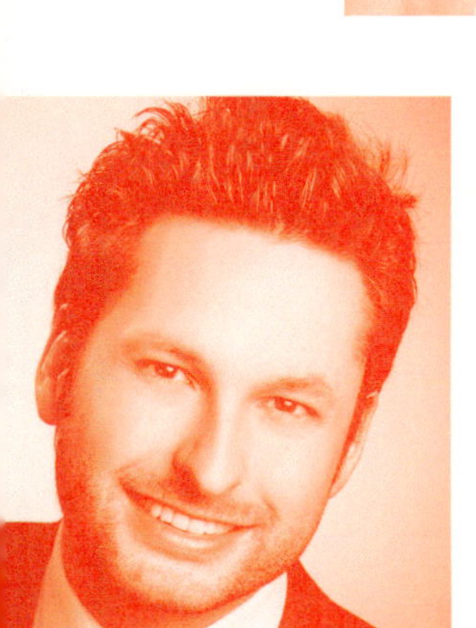
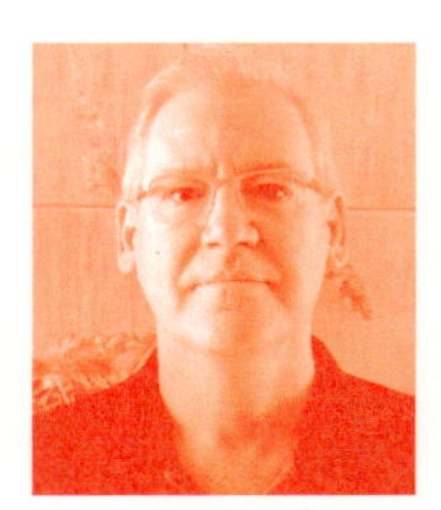
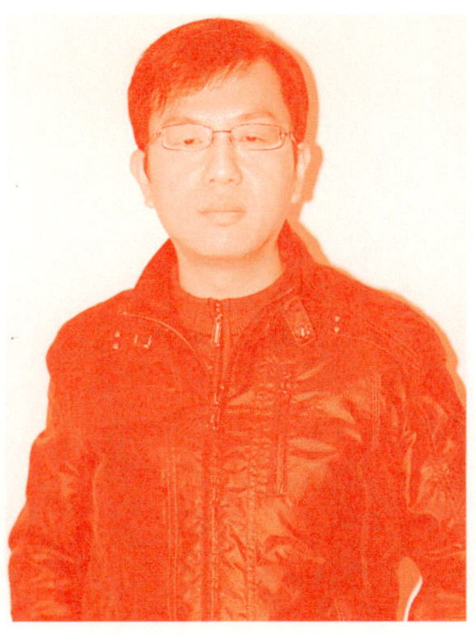

IntechOpen

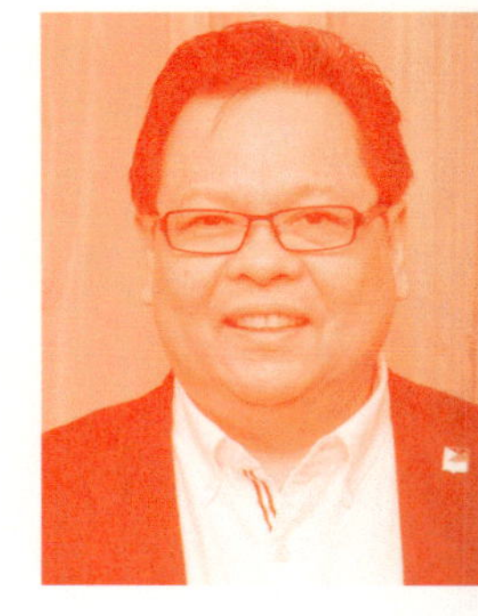
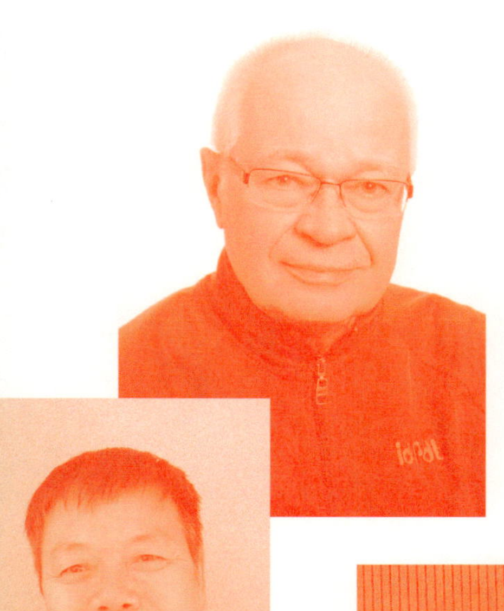
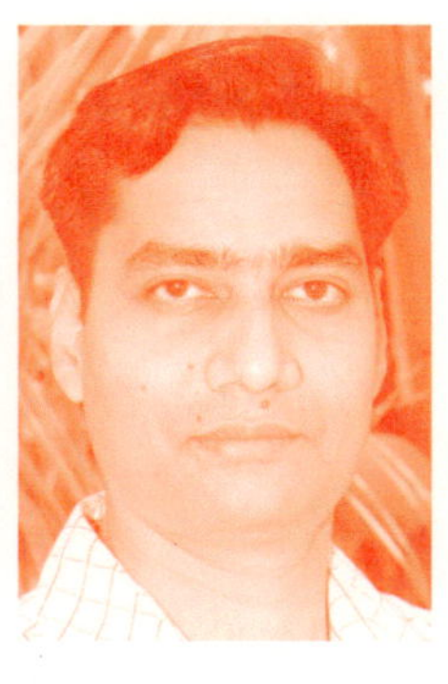
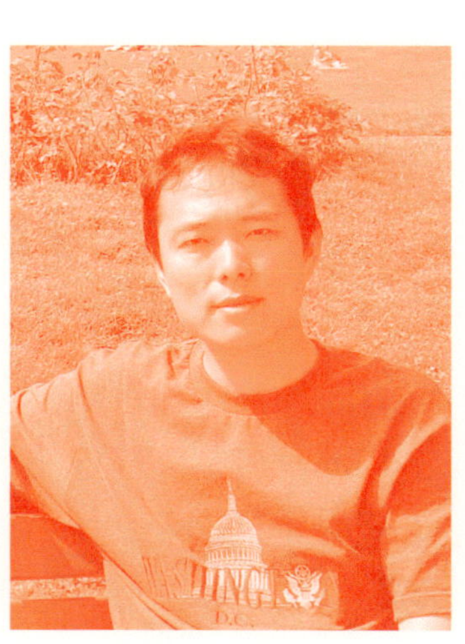
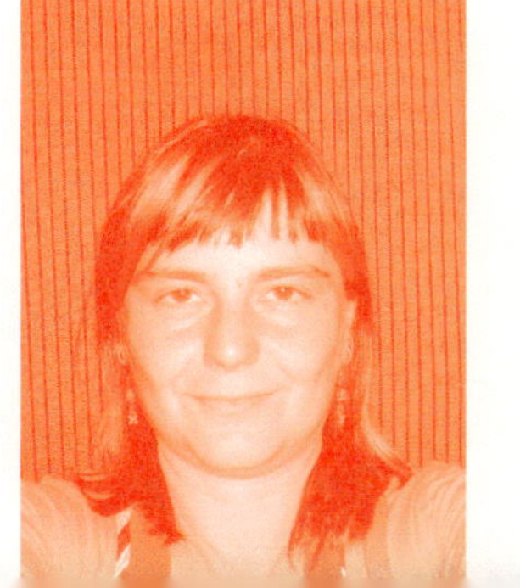

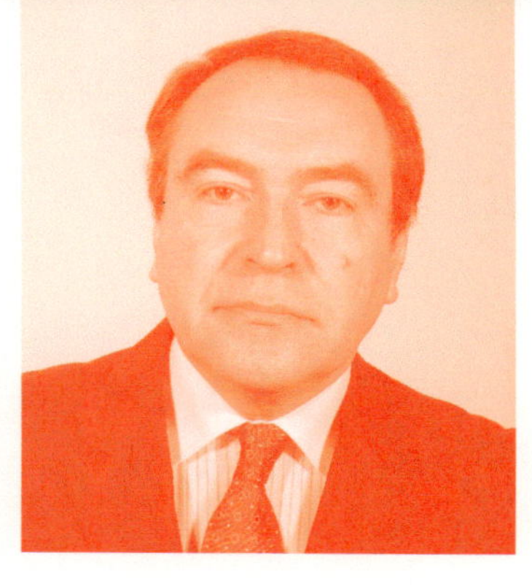
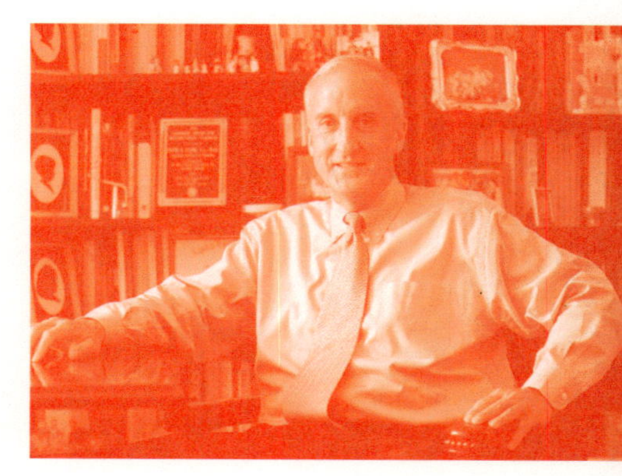
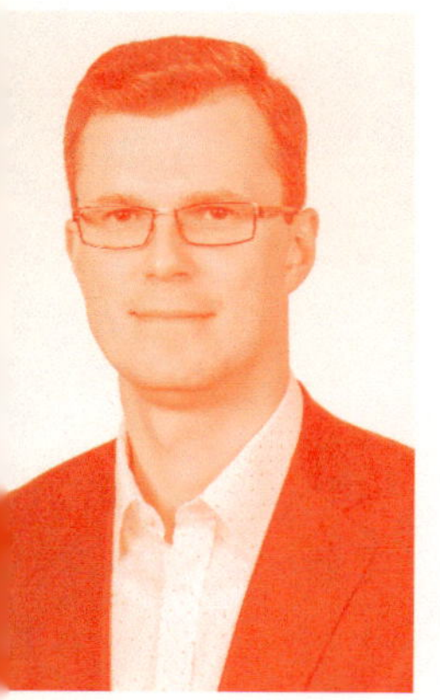
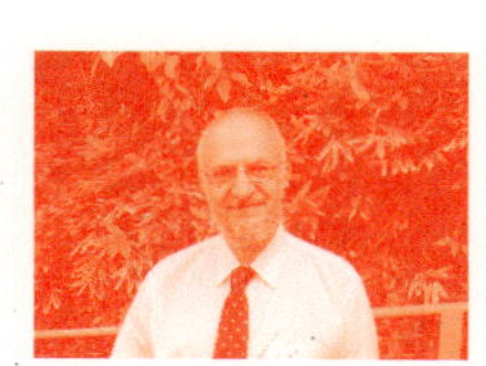
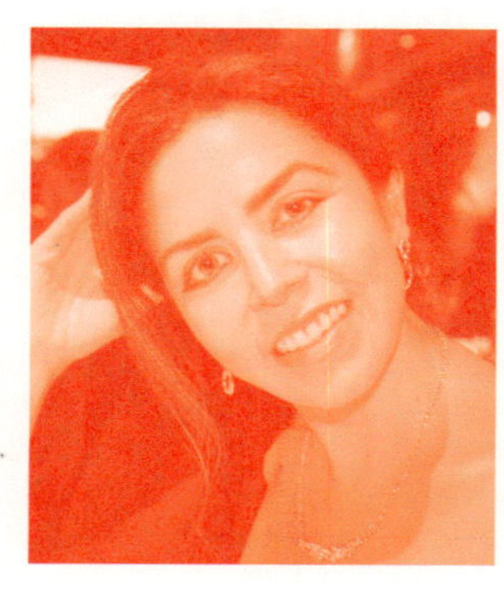

Supporting open minds since 2005

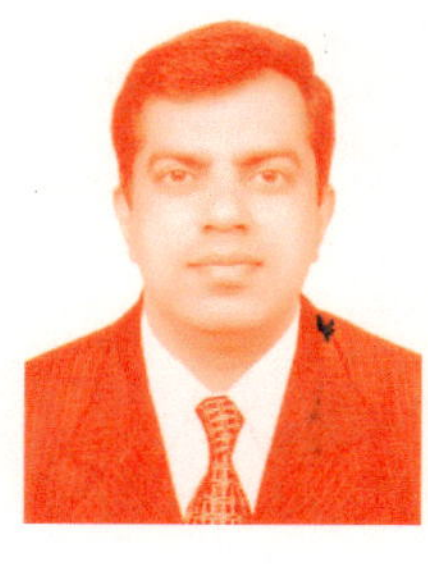
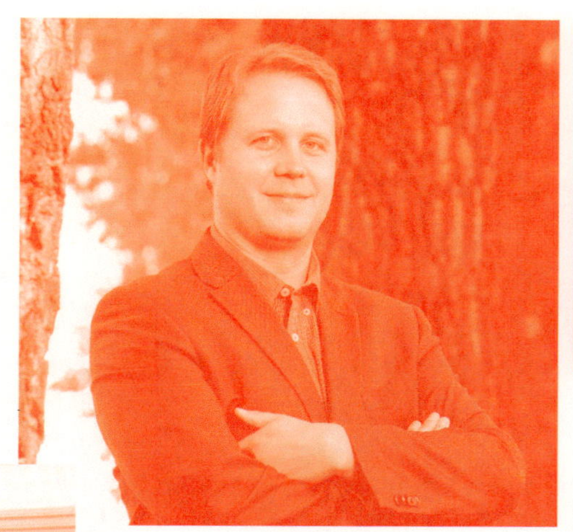
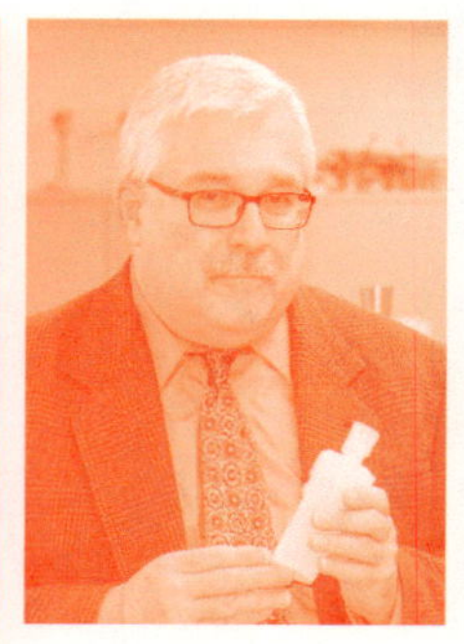
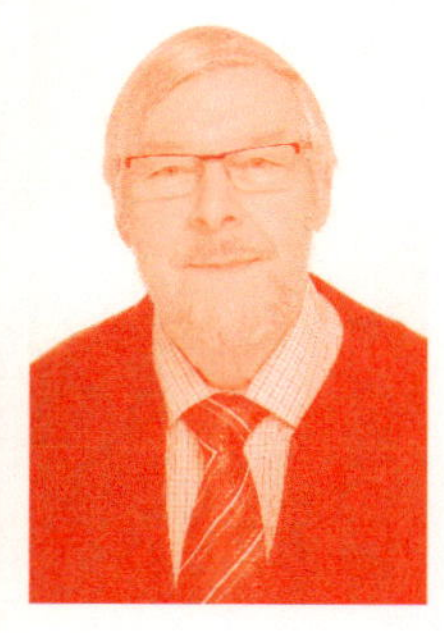
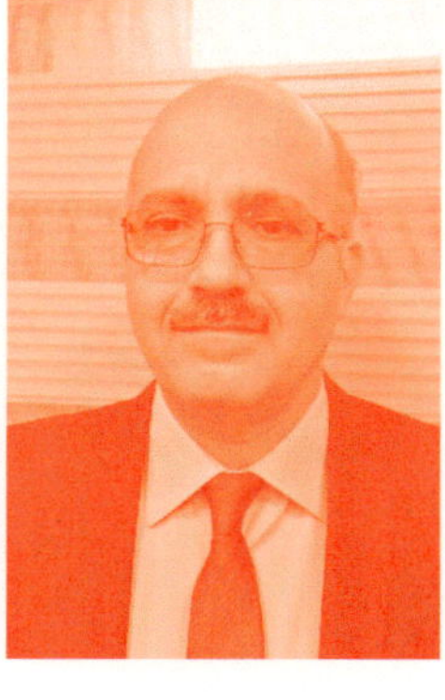
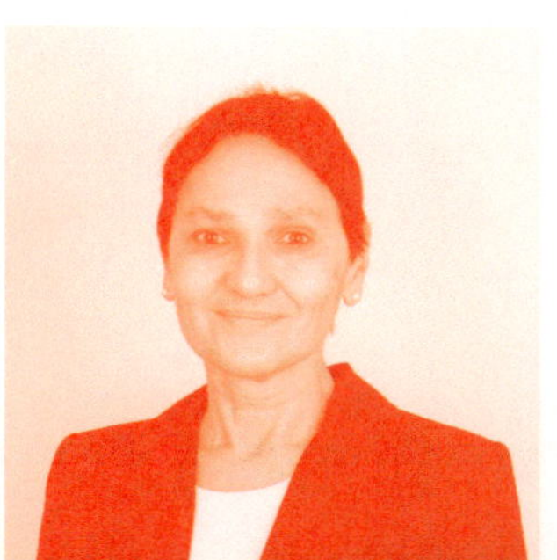
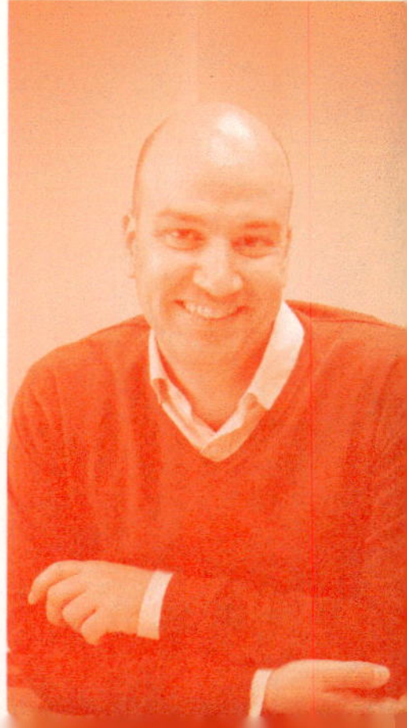

Neutrophils
http://dx.doi.org/10.5772/intechopen.73927
Edited by Maitham Khajah

Contributors
Elaine Cruz Rosas, Mariana C. Souza, Carlos Rosales, Eileen Uribe-Querol, Galina Chudilova, Irina Nesterova, Ludmila Lomtatidze, Svetlana Kovaleva, Tatyana Rusinova, Robert Allen, Maitham Khajah

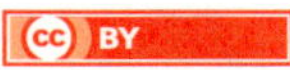

First published in London, United Kingdom, 2019 by IntechOpen
IntechOpen is the global imprint of INTECHOPEN LIMITED, registered in England and Wales, registration number: 11086078, The Shard, 25th floor, 32 London Bridge Street
London, SE19SG - United Kingdom
Printed in Croatia

British Library Cataloguing-in-Publication Data
A catalogue record for this book is available from the British Library

Additional hard copies can be obtained from orders@intechopen.com

Neutrophils
Edited by Maitham Khajah
p. cm.
Print ISBN 978-1-78985-285-1
Online ISBN 978-1-78985-286-8

For EU product safety concerns:
IN TECH d.o.o., Prolaz Marije Krucifikse Kozulić 3, 51000 Rijeka, Croatia, info@intechopen.com or visit our website at intechopen.com.

Meet the editor

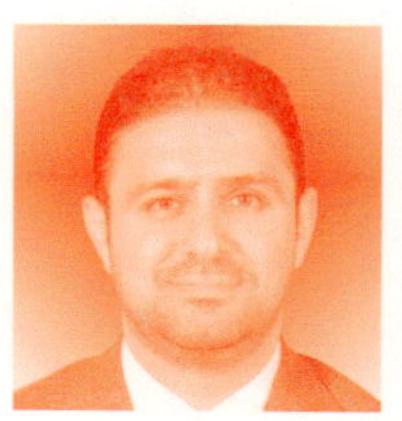

Dr. Maitham Khajah completed his BPharm degree from the Faculty of Pharmacy, Kuwait University, in 2003 and obtained his PhD degree in December 2009 from the University of Calgary, Canada (Gastrointestinal Science and Immunology). He was employed as an assistant professor in 2010 and was recently promoted to associate professor at Kuwait University, Faculty of Pharmacy, Department of Pharmacology and Therapeutics. He is currently the Chairman of the Department of Pharmacology and Therapeutics. His research interest is to study new molecular targets for the treatment of inflammatory bowel disease and breast cancer. He has supervised many students for the MSc Molecular Biology and Pharmaceutical Sciences Programs, College of Graduate Studies, Kuwait University. He joined Kuwait University in 2010, and received various grants such as PI and Co-I. He was awarded the Best Young Researcher award by Kuwait University, Research Sector, for the Year 2013–2014.

Contents

Preface

Polymorphnuclear cells (or neutrophils) are the most abundant type of immune cells in the blood and play an integral role in innate and adaptive immunity towards various infectious and non-infectious triggers. These cells have the capability to perform various effector functions such as phagocytosis, degranulation, motility/chemotaxis, and the recently discovered function called neutrophil extracellular traps formation and subsequent microbial killing. *Neutrophils* provides recent evidence regarding the various properties of these immune cells in relation to various disease conditions aimed at future therapeutic targets.

Chapter 1 (Introductory Chapter: Background Summary Regarding Neutrophils) briefly discusses the basic effector functions of neutrophils, which provide the basis for the upcoming chapters in the book.

Chapter 2 (Cannabinoid Receptors as Regulators of Neutrophil Activity in Inflammatory Diseases) discusses how cannabinoids (binding through their receptors: CR-1 and -2) can modulate various activities of neutrophils, and act as a therapeutic target for various neutrophil-related inflammatory (e.g. arthritis, ischemic diseases, and colitis) and infectious (e.g. sepsis and mycobacterial infection) conditions.

Chapter 3 (Neutrophil Activation by Antibody Receptors) discusses the role of neutrophils in the adaptive immune response through their interactions with immunoglobulins (mainly IgG) secreted by B-cells. The main types of FcγRs located on neutrophils and how particular FcγRs can activate various signaling pathways to promote unique effector cell functions are also discussed in this chapter.

Chapter 4 (Remodeling of Phenotype $CD16^{+}CD11b^{+}$ Neutrophilic Granulocytes in Acute Viral and Acute Bacterial Infections) discusses the different expression patterns of the membrane receptors CD16 and CD11b in normal and pathological conditions such as in patients with acute viral and acute bacterial tonsillitis. The differential membranous expression profile of these receptors on the neutrophils may help in the early-stage diagnosis of these conditions.

Chapter 5 (Essence of Reducing Equivalent Transfer Powering Neutrophil Oxidative Microbicide Action and Chemiluminescence) discusses the physics of the NADPH oxidase system and the detection of the generated reactive oxygen species using various chemiluminigenic probes for circulating blood neutrophils, which can aid in *in vivo* state of host inflammatory activation.

We hope that the recent evidence described in this book provides a better understanding of the role of this important immune cell in various disease conditions and forms the basis for future research activities aimed at providing better therapeutic approaches to treat various disease conditions.

Dr. Maitham Khajah, BPharm, PhD
Associate Professor and Chairman,
Department of Pharmacology and Therapeutics,
Faculty of Pharmacy, Kuwait University,
Kuwait

Chapter 1

Introductory Chapter: Background Summary Regarding Neutrophils

Maitham Khajah

1. Neutrophils: important immune cells in health and diseas

Neutrophils are key players in the innate and the adaptive immunity and contribute to the pathogenesis of various infectious and noninfectious conditions. These cells have the capability of performing various effector functions and therefore are considered an important therapeutic target for many conditions. They are considered the fastest immune cells in our body and the first to arrive to the inflammatory site. This occurs in response to a wide variety of chemoattractive agents, such as CXC chemokines [keratinocyte-derived cytokine (KC), macrophage inflammatory protein-2 (MIP-2)], lipid mediators [leukotriene B_4 (LTB_4) and platelet-activating factor (PAF)], the complement split product (C5a), and the bacterial toxin formyl-met-leu-phe (fMLP)] [1]. Neutrophils use different intracellular signaling pathways in their migrative behavior which are dependent on the type of chemoattractant they encounter [1–3].

These immune cells also play an important role in the recognition of various pathogens through specific cell surface and cytoplasmic receptors including toll-like receptors (TLRs) and nucleotide oligomerization domains (NODs). In addition, they can also recognize opsonized particles through the complement receptors and mediate antibody-dependent cell cytotoxicity (ADCC) through their interaction with immunoglobulin receptors [4–6]. They can also mediate microbial killing through oxygen-dependent and oxygen-independent mechanisms. In response to various ligands, this results in a dramatic increase in oxygen consumption due to the activation of nicotinamide adenine dinucleotide phosphate (NADPH) oxidase system leading to the generation of various reactive oxygen (e.g., superoxide anion radical) [7] and nitrogen (through nitric oxide synthase; NOS) intermediates [8]. This can not only aid in microbial killing but also contribute to the pathogenesis of various inflammatory and cancerous conditions (through the generation of peroxynitrite). The non-oxidative arm of neutrophil killing is mediated through the action of antimicrobial peptides and proteases present in various compartments of azurophilic (primary), specific (secondary), gelatinase, and secretary granules [9–13].

This book provides recent evidence regarding the role of cannabinoid receptors (CR-1 and CR-2) and different subtypes of the immunoglobulin receptor FcγRs in the pathogenesis, diagnosis, and treatment of various diseases of infectious and noninfectious origin. Furthermore, the differential expression pattern of CD16 + CD11b + receptors on the surface of neutrophils and their role in the diagnosis of acute viral and bacterial infections will also be highlighted. Finally, the utility of using different chemiluminigenic probes for the detection of NADPH activity for the circulating blood neutrophils and their role in determining the in vivo state of host inflammatory activation will be highlighted in this book.

IntechOpen

Author details

Maitham Khajah
Department of Pharmacology and Therapeutics, Faculty of Pharmacy, Kuwait University, Kuwait

*Address all correspondence to: maitham@hsc.edu.kw

References

[1] Heit B, Tavener S, Raharjo E, Kubes P. An intracellular signaling hierarchy determines direction of migration in opposing chemotactic gradients. The Journal of Cell Biology. 2002;**159**(1): 91-102. Epub 2002 Oct 7

[2] Khajah M, Andonegui G, Chan R, Craig AW, Greer PA, McCafferty DM. Fer kinase limits neutrophil chemotaxis toward end target chemoattractants. Journal of Immunology. 2013;**190**(5):2208-2216

[3] Heit B, Robbins SM, Downey CM, Guan Z, Colarusso P, Miller BJ, et al. PTEN functions to 'prioritize' chemotactic cues and prevent 'distraction' in migrating neutrophils. Nature Immunology. 2008;**9**(7):743-752. DOI: ni.1623 [pii]10.1038/ni.1623

[4] Hayashi F, Means TK, Luster AD. Toll-like receptors stimulate human neutrophil function. Blood. 2003;**102**(7):2660-2669

[5] Lee WL, Harrison RE, Grinstein S. Phagocytosis by neutrophils. Microbes and Infection. 2003;**5**(14):1299-1306

[6] Stuart LM, Ezekowitz RA. Phagocytosis: Elegant complexity. Immunity. 2005;**22**(5):539-550

[7] McCord JM, Fridovich I. The biology and pathology of oxygen radicals. Annals of Internal Medicine. 1978;**89**(1):122-127

[8] Kruidenier L, Kuiper I, Lamers CB, Verspaget HW. Intestinal oxidative damage in inflammatory bowel disease: Semi-quantification, localization, and association with mucosal antioxidants. The Journal of Pathology. 2003;**201**(1):28-36. DOI: 10.1002/path.1409

[9] Belaaouaj A, McCarthy R, Baumann M, Gao Z, Ley TJ, Abraham SN, et al. Mice lacking neutrophil elastase reveal impaired host defense against gram negative bacterial sepsis. Nature Medicine. 1998;**4**(5):615-618

[10] Reeves EP, Lu H, Jacobs HL, Messina CG, Bolsover S, Gabella G, et al. Killing activity of neutrophils is mediated through activation of proteases by K+ flux. Nature. 2002;**416**(6878):291-297

[11] Tkalcevic J, Novelli M, Phylactides M, Iredale JP, Segal AW, Roes J. Impaired immunity and enhanced resistance to endotoxin in the absence of neutrophil elastase and cathepsin G. Immunity. 2000;**12**(2):201-210

[12] Pham CT. Neutrophil serine proteases: Specific regulators of inflammation. Nature Reviews. Immunology. 2006;**6**(7):541-550

[13] Faurschou M, Borregaard N. Neutrophil granules and secretory vesicles in inflammation. Microbes and Infection. 2003;**5**(14):1317-1327

Chapter 2

Cannabinoid Receptors as Regulators of Neutrophil Activity in Inflammatory Diseases

Mariana Conceição Souza and Elaine Cruz Rosas

Abstract

Cannabinoids are compounds present in *Cannabis sativa* (phytocannabinoids), endogenously produced (endocannabinoids) or synthesized, that bind to G protein-coupled receptors named cannabinoid receptors B1 and B2. They were first described as psychotropic compounds; however, cannabinoids are also potent immunoregulatory agents. Cannabinoids can modulate neutrophil activity in sterile and infectious inflammatory diseases. Concerning sterile inflammatory diseases as arthritis, ischemic diseases, and colitis, the use of CB2 agonist impairs the intracellular signaling pathways involved in the production of inflammatory mediators and expression of adhesion molecules. As a consequence, neutrophils did not release metalloproteinases either to adhere to endothelial cells, resulting in reduced tissue damage. A similar anti-inflammatory CB2 agonist mechanism of action in sepsis and mycobacterial infection models is observed. However, it is not clear if inflammation resolution promoted by cannabinoid treatment during infection is also related to microbial viability. Despite the growing literature showing the effects of cannabinoids on neutrophils, there are still some gaps that should be filled before proposing cannabinoid-based drugs to treat neutrophil-dependent diseases.

Keywords: cannabinoid agonist, inflammation, infection, endocannabinoids, phytocannabinoids, synthetic cannabinoids

1. Introduction

Neutrophils have been classically recognized as the most relevant cell during acute inflammatory responses and, more recently, in chronic inflammation [1]. On the one hand, neutrophils produce bactericidal molecules and coordinate the accumulation of pro-resolving cells. On the other hand, neutrophil over activation leads to tissue damage. In this context, several approaches have been proposed to regulate the accumulation and the activity of neutrophils in pathological conditions.

In parallel, the findings concerning the importance of the endocannabinoid system as the endogenous immunoregulatory mechanism raise questions on how it could be therapeutically used to treat inflammatory diseases. In this chapter, we discuss how the endocannabinoid system can be used to modulate the activity of neutrophils in sterile and infectious inflammatory diseases.

2. Cannabinoid system

Cannabis sativa (marijuana) is one of the oldest plants that produced psychoactive effects on humans. In addition, it has been used in medicine in controlling pain, convulsion, inflammation, and asthma [2, 3]. Cannabinoids are a group of lipophilic and pharmacologically active compounds present in *C. sativa*. The first component from cannabis identified was the tetrahydrocannabinol (Δ9-THC) and and, as other cannabinoids, binds to G protein-coupled receptors (GPCRs) named cannabinoid receptors [4, 5].

Cannabinoid receptor agonists are responsible for several biological effects, such as analgesic, antiemetic, antitumor, and anti-inflammatory [6–13], and are classified into three groups based on their origin: endogenous cannabinoids (endocannabinoids—**Figure 1a** and **b**), phytocannabinoids (**Figure 1c** and **d**), and synthetic cannabinoids (**Figure 1e** and **f**) [5].

Endocannabinoids (eCBs) are eicosanoids derived from polyunsaturated chain fatty acids, such as arachidonic acid, and comprise amides, esters, and ether [14]. Anandamide (AEA) was the first endocannabinoid described in the mammalian

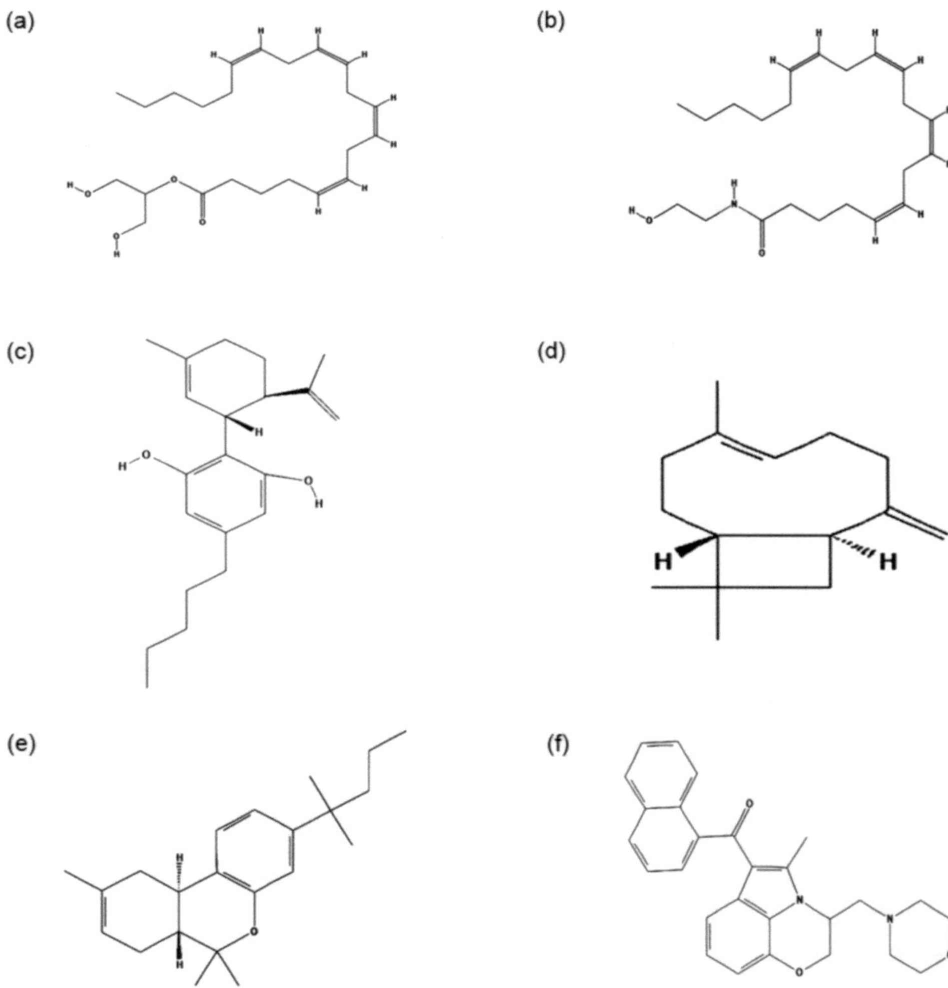

Figure 1.
Chemical structure of some representatives of the cannabinoid agonists. (a) 2-AG, (b) AEA, (c) cannabidiol, (d) β-caryophyllene, (e) JWH-133, and (f) WIN 55212-2.

brain and other tissues [15], followed by 2-arachidonoylglycerol (2-AG) [16, 17]. The AEA and 2-AG represent the major substances of this class. The eCBs together with the cannabinoid receptors and the enzymes that regulate their biosynthesis and degradation constitute the "endocannabinoid system" [18]. Beyond the well-known psychotropic effects, the endocannabinoid system plays an essential immunomodulatory role by modulating the release of cytokines and on acute or chronical diseases through two main ways, neuro- and immunomodulation [19, 20].

The group of phytocannabinoids consists of active substances initially extracted from *Cannabis sativa*, whose pharmacological activity is associated with the terpene phenolic class. Phytocannabinoids are classified into two groups: psychoactive cannabinoids, such as Δ9-THC, and non-psychoactive such as cannabidiol and cannabinol [21, 22]. More recently, other molecules have been isolated from different plant species, which exert effects through cannabinoid receptors, such as the alkylamides derived from *Echinacea angustifolia* and *Otanthus maritimus* and sesquiterpene, as β-caryophyllene, found in some plant species from *Copaifera* genus [23–27].

The characterization of the chemical structure of Δ9-THC and endocannabinoids allowed the development of synthetic cannabinoids. From THC, it was possible to synthesize several compounds that have similar chemical structures with different levels of affinity for cannabinoid receptors [5, 28]. Synthetic cannabinoids have been used as a pharmacological tool for *in vivo* or *in vitro* studies to explore the therapeutic potential of the cannabinoid system. However, it has already been described that metabolites form dipyrone and paracetamol exert its analgesic effects by inhibiting endocannabinoid biosynthesis and binding of cannabinoid receptors, respectively [29].

The cannabinoid receptors CB1 and CB2 are the main receptors of the cannabinoid system. Both belong to the family of GPCRs, specifically inhibitory G protein (Gi) [30]. The binding of agonists to cannabinoid receptors inhibits adenylate cyclase (AC) and modulates activation of different members of the MAPK family, including ERK1/ERK2, p38, and JNK1/2 (**Figure 2**) [30–37]. By inhibiting AC, the reduction of the second messenger cyclic adenosine monophosphate (cAMP) leads to the opening of rectifying potassium channels. CB1 also mediates the inhibition of N-type and P/Q-type calcium currents [22, 38]. Besides CB1 and CB2, the existence of a third cannabinoid receptor (CB3) has been suggested [39], and there are two orphan G protein-coupled receptors (GPCRs) which overlap with CB1 and CB2, named GPR18 and GPR55 [40]. In addition to activation via GPCRs, cannabinoids can perform their actions by activating PPARs, including PPARγ [41–43].

CB1 is expressed in the central nervous system, especially by neurons [44] and modulates physiological processes, such as motor behavior, learning, memory and cognition, and pain perception [45]. This receptor is associated with the psychotropic effects of cannabinoid agonists, such as THC [46, 47].

CB2 is the peripheral receptor for cannabinoid agonists. It is mainly expressed in immune tissues such as the spleen and thymus as well as in blood cell subpopulations such as CD4 and CD8 lymphocytes, neutrophils, monocytes, natural killer (NK) cells, and B lymphocytes [47]. Nevertheless, CB2 is also found at low levels in neuronal and nonneuronal cells of the brain, but it does not produce psychoactive effects [47–49].

The CB2 expression intensity in immune cells depends on cell populations and activation state [50, 51]. Macrophages from different tissues increase CB2 expression after stimulation with interferon (IFN)-γ, which suggests that macrophages activated during an inflammatory process are more sensitive to the action of cannabinoid agonists than those in the resting state [52]. The first evidence that cannabinoids might modulate cytokine production was in the mid-1980s when murine

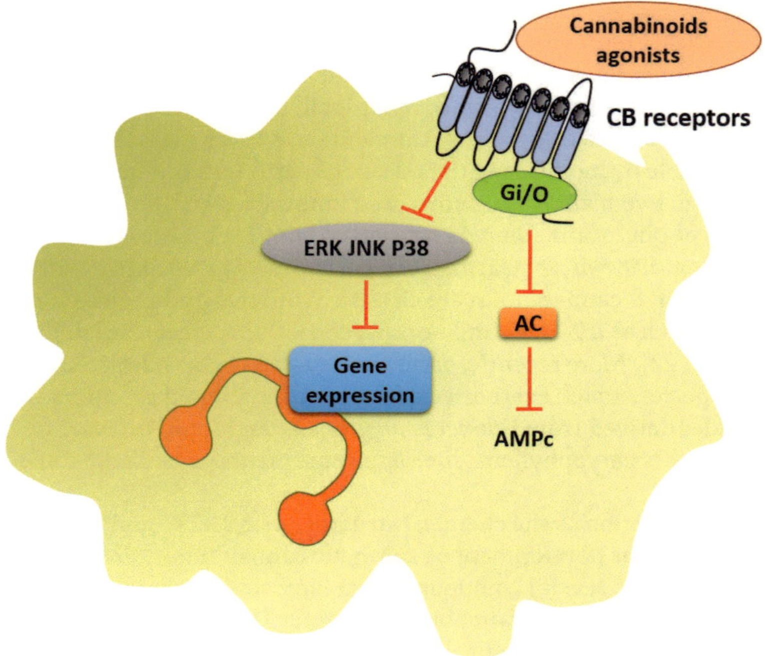

Figure 2.
Neutrophil activated expresses cannabinoid receptors (CB receptors). The cannabinoid receptors CB1 and CB2 belong to the family of GPCRs, specifically inhibitory G protein (Gi/o). The binding of agonists to cannabinoid receptors inhibits the activation of different members of the MAPK family (ERK1/2, p38, and JNK1/2), gene expression, as well as reduces cyclic adenosine monophosphate (cAMP) levels by inhibiting adenylate cyclase (AC) activity.

cells treated with agonist cannabinoid reduced the levels of type I interferons (IFN-α and IFN-β) after stimulation with LPS or polyinosinic-polycytidylic acid (polyI:C). Many subsequent studies have shown that cannabinoids inhibited the production of cytokines in innate and adaptive immune responses, both in animal models and in human cell cultures (to review [53]). In such a way, CB2 has become an important target, especially in inflammatory conditions. The CB2 receptor modulates immune cell functions, both *in vitro* and in animal models of inflammatory diseases. In this context, some studies have reported that mice lacking the CB2 receptor have an exacerbated inflammatory phenotype (to review [19]). Besides, CB2 agonists have an inhibitory effect on leukocyte migration and in the production of pro-inflammatory mediators *in vivo* and *in vitro*, showing a high anti-inflammatory potential [54]. Due to the lack of psychotropic effects, CB2 agonists are considered a promising therapeutic strategy for the treatment of chronic inflammatory diseases. Preclinical studies showed the action of CB2 agonists on different experimental models of inflammation, such as colitis, arthritis, cerebral ischemia, and sepsis [10, 53, 55–59], and in these studies, they showed that the action of CB2 agonists modulated the neutrophil activity.

3. Neutrophils, cannabinoid system, inflammation, and infection

3.1 Neutrophils and cannabinoid system

Neutrophils play a crucial role in inflammatory processes, which are present in the pathology of different diseases. The neutrophil recruitment to the inflammatory site is an essential stage in the inflammatory responses; these cells are released from the bone marrow to the periphery immediately after the first signal of inflammation. The mobilization of neutrophils from the bone marrow is conducted by the hematopoietic cytokine granulocyte colony-stimulating factor (G-CSF), which mobilizes neutrophils indirectly by shifting the balance between ligands to CXCR4 (CXCL12) and CXCR2 (CXCL1 and CXCL2) [60]. Neutrophil-active chemoattractant, as chemokines CXCL1 and CXCL2, is produced and released within the bone marrow and in inflamed tissue. In this context, chemokines from inflamed foci might make their way to the bone marrow and modulate neutrophil egress. Thus, CXCL1 and CXCL2 can act locally by inducing neutrophil recruitment from blood to peripheral tissue and systemically by inducing neutrophil mobilization from the bone marrow to the bloodstream [61].

Once in the peripheral blood, neutrophils can be rapidly recruited into inflamed or infected tissues. A panel of diverse stimuli, especially pathogen-associated molecular patterns (PAMPs) and damage-associated molecular patterns (DAMPs), activates macrophages, mast cells, or stromal cells to produce and release pro-inflammatory mediators as interleukin (IL)-1β, tumor necrosis factor (TNF), CXCL8, CXCL1, CXCL2, and lipid mediators, such as leukotriene B_4 (LTB_4) and endocannabinoids [61, 62]. In inflammatory loci, neutrophils find antigen, molecules, and/or immune complexes that trigger different actions, such as phagocytosis, production of reactive oxygen species (ROS), and release of enzyme-rich granules (as collagenases, gelatinases, neutrophil myeloperoxidase (MPO), and elastase [63]). Neutrophils enter the tissue through surface molecules which interact with vascular endothelial cells. This process is accompanied by a regulated rearrangement of the cytoskeleton of neutrophils that lead to actin polymerization [64], which is mainly governed by members of the Rho family GTPases including RhoA, Rac1, and Cdc42 [65].

Concerning cannabinoid receptor expression, it was observed that neutrophil from healthy donors expresses low levels of CB2 [66]. In addition, it was shown that the CB2 receptor plays a crucial role in neutrophil differentiation, and it has been implicated in the development of leukemia [67, 68].

The role of the cannabinoid system in neutrophil migration is controversial. The activation of CB2 receptors by 2-AG did not induce polarization and migration of human blood neutrophils [69]. However, pretreatment of neutrophils with 2-AG inhibited the fMLP- and CXCL8-induced migration without affecting the polarization of the cells [69]. In contrast, McHugh and coworkers showed that 2-AG does not inhibit the migration of human neutrophils toward fMLP and does not show chemotactic effects by itself [70]. Furthermore, Balenga and coworkers showed that 2-AG induces migration of neutrophils toward inflammatory sites, through cross talk with activated GPR55 [62].

Despite the uncertainty regarding the involvement of CB2 agonist with the neutrophil migration and action, some studies show that there is a relationship between neutrophils and cannabinoid system in the pathogenesis of inflammatory or infection diseases (**Table 1**). In the next section, we will discuss the cannabinoid system and its action on the neutrophil participation in inflammatory and infection conditions [54, 62, 69–85].

3.2 Neutrophils, cannabinoid system, and inflammation

The action of CB2 agonists on their receptors impairs the secretion of pro-inflammatory cytokines and chemokines and reduces the recruitment of neutrophils. As discussed previously, neutrophils play a significant role in inflammatory diseases, including acute, chronic, autoimmune, infectious, and noninfectious conditions. The relation between neutrophil and cannabinoid system in inflammatory disease was discussed in this section.

Drugs	Mechanism of action on neutrophils	Reference
Endocannabinoids		
N-arachidonoyl-ethanolamine (AEA)	Decreases neutrophil migration in vitro	70
	Decreases neutrophil migration in vivo	71
2-arachidonoylgycerol (2-AG)	Decreases neutrophil migration in vitro	69
	Increases neutrophil motility	62, 72
Phytocannabinoids		
cannabidiol	Neutrophil deactivation in vitro	70, 73, 74
	Decreases neutrophil migration in vivo	74, 75, 76, 77
Delta 9-tetrahydrocannabidiol (THC)	Decreases neutrophil migration in vivo	77, 78, 79
beta-caryophyllene		
	Decreases neutrophil migration in vivo	
		54, 80, 81, 82
	Decreases neutrophil migration in vitro	83
Synthetic cannabinoid		
HU-308	Decreases neutrophil migration in vivo	77
JWH-133	Neutrophil deactivation in vitro	84
WIN55212-2	Decreases neutrophil migration in vivo and in vitro	71

Table 1.
Cannabinoid agonists, which exert action on neutrophils.

Increased macro- and microscopic colon damage scores, a high number of macrophage and neutrophil and MPO activity, characterizes experimental colitis. The activation of CB receptors by their ligands produces a protective effect in experimental colitis by decreasing prostaglandin, ROS and nitric oxide production, and reduction of leukocyte accumulation as neutrophils, resulting in diminished of colon tissue inflammation. Besides, mice lacking functional CB receptors are less resistant to colon inflammation than wild-type animals [53, 86]. The synthetic non-psychotropic cannabinoids as JWH-133, cannabinoid from the plant as cannabigerol [87] and β-caryophyllene [54], and synthetic atypical cannabinoid O-1602 (non-CB1 and CB2 ligands) [88] have been able to inhibit neutrophil recruitment in colitis models. Thus, during inflammation, the CB2 receptor activation by endocannabinoids or synthetic cannabinoid provides a mechanism for the reestablishment of regular GI transit (to review [89]).

Neutrophils are also essential cells in the development of arthritis. Neutrophils are abundant in inflamed joints, and these cells are essential to the initiation and progression of rheumatoid arthritis (RA). Neutrophil effector mechanisms include the release of pro-inflammatory cytokines, reactive oxygen and nitrogen species

(ROS and RNS), and granules containing derivative enzymes, which can cause further damage to the tissue and amplify the inflammatory response [90]. In such way, it has already been described that in RA there is an increase of CB2 expression and elevated endocannabinoid levels, observed in the synovial tissue and fluid from a patient with this disease [91]. Synovial fibroblasts and macrophages are mainly responsible for endocannabinoid production. These cells also are essential in the production of chemokines (CXCR1 or 2 ligands, such as CXCL8), the C5a fragment of the complement system, and LTB_4 which are responsible for neutrophil mobilization to the synovial cavity [61]. In this context, the activation of CB2 receptors inhibits the production of pro-inflammatory mediators, like chemokines, which reduces the leukocyte migration, like neutrophils, to the synovial cavity and metalloproteinase release [92]. Moreover, the activation of CB2 receptors inhibits IL-1β-induced activation of extracellular signal-regulated kinases 1 and 2 and p38 mitogen-activated protein kinase in RA fibroblast [92].

The role of cannabinoid in neutrophils was also studied in ischemic models. Endocannabinoids act via the CB2 receptor in the modulation of the inflammatory response and myocardial remodeling after infarction. CB2 receptor plays an essential role in the formation of infarction border zone, collagen deposition, and organization of stable scar during remodeling. Duerr and coworkers [93] showed increased numbers of neutrophils in the heart ischemic area of CB2 receptor-deficient (Cnr2−/−) mice when compared with healthy mice. These results suggest that CB2 receptor modulates neutrophil migration to inflammatory infarction site [93]. In accordance, activation of the cannabinoid CB2 receptor by JWH-133 protects against atherosclerotic plaque formation and may also decrease neutrophil MMP-9 release, which reduces the vulnerability of ischemic stroke plaque in arteries. Together, the studies suggest that CB2 agonists represent a promising anti-atherosclerotic treatment [84].

Even though CB1 is the most prominent receptor in the CNS, CB2 modulates neuroinflammation. CB2 activation by JWH-133 reduced the number of neutrophils in the ischemic brain. Furthermore, CB2 activation *in vitro* inhibits adherence of neutrophils to brain endothelial cells. JWH-133 also interfered with the migration of neutrophils induced by the endogenous chemokine CXCL2 through activation of the MAP kinase p38. This effect on neutrophils is probably responsible for the neuroprotection mediated by JWH-133 [56].

3.3 Neutrophils, cannabinoid system, and infection

The relation between neutrophil and infection is well established [94]. On one hand, the exacerbation of neutrophil activation could lead to tissue damage. On the other hand, neutrophils control microorganism growth. In this context, it is essential to study the effect of cannabinoids on neutrophils during infections and evaluate if and how the cannabinoid system modulates neutrophil activity.

The interest in the relationship among cannabinoids and infections exists since the 1960s when studies regarding "hippie subculture" observed the increase of sexually transmitted infections by marijuana consumers [95]. By this time, the studies focused on consumer behavior and how it could increase susceptibility to infections but did not evaluate the effect of cannabinoids on host response to infections [96]. Nowadays, it is known that endocannabinoid system regulates and is regulated by host microbiota, a balance that protects the host from the infection-triggered inflammatory response [29]. However, the increase of studies showing the immunoregulatory role of the endocannabinoid system raises questions about if cannabinoids could modulate microbial viability and/or neutrophil response during infections.

Studies concerning the modulation of neutrophil activity by cannabinoids during infections are mostly addressed to experimental bacterial infection as sepsis model. Neutrophil activity during experimental sepsis is well characterized in studies *in vivo* (to review [97–99]). By using LPS sepsis model, Smith and coworkers showed that treatment with cannabinoid receptor agonists reduced the migration of neutrophils in the peritoneal cavity by inhibiting neutrophil chemoattractant production [59]. The authors conclude that CB2 was responsible for impairing neutrophil migration. In accordance, studies performed in CB2-deficient mice submitted to sepsis induced by cecal ligation and puncture showed increased production of neutrophil chemotactic chemokines and increased numbers of neutrophil in the bone marrow and lung tissue. Interestingly, despite the increase in neutrophil numbers, neutrophils from CB2-deficient mice were not able to activate the MAPK pathway neither control bacterial load [57, 100]. Furthermore, in mycobacteria model of infection, it was observed that CB2 agonism impairs neutrophil adhesion to endothelial cells probably by inhibiting actin polymerization [83].

There are few and controverting data concerning CB1 effects on neutrophils during infection. Leite-Avalca and coworkers showed that CB1 antagonist given to mice submitted to CLP increased the survival rate but not change neutrophil accumulation in the peritoneal cavity [101]. Nevertheless, Kianian and coworkers showed that antagonism of CB1 reduced the adhesion of leukocytes to intestinal submucosal venules [102]. It is noteworthy that in the sepsis model, the activation of CB1 increases the systemic arterial pressure and the flow and decreases the arterial oxygenation; however, it decreases the inflammatory cytokine production [103, 104]. In such a way, an indirect effect of CB1 on leukocyte behavior during sepsis cannot be ruled out.

The results regarding the immunomodulatory effects of cannabinoids in infection are in accordance with the host-directed therapy approach that aims to activate protective responses against microbes in addition to antimicrobial therapy [105]. However, it should be mentioned that antibiotics perturb gut microflora, which could result in the endocannabinoid system unbalance and, thus, in neuropsychiatric disorders [29]. Indeed, further studies are necessary to propose to activate the endocannabinoid system, especially the CB2 pathway, during infections.

4. Conclusion

An increasing amount of data concerning the immunoregulatory role of cannabinoids, especially the CB2 agonists, has been raising the interest in developing new therapeutic strategies for inflammatory diseases. It is already known that the mechanism of action of well-established anti-inflammatory drugs, like paracetamol, depends on the activation of the endocannabinoid system [29]. However, despite all studies showing that cannabinoids can modulate neutrophil biology, there is a long way to go to achieve cannabinoid-based drugs to treat neutrophil-dependent diseases such as arthritis and infection-induced acute lung injury.

Acknowledgements

The authors express their gratitude to Luana Barbosa Correa at the Laboratory of Applied Pharmacology (Farmanguinhos, FIOCRUZ) for her support in drawing **Figure 2**. This work was supported by grants from the Brazilian Council for Scientific and Technological Development (CNPq), Carlos Chagas Filho, Rio de Janeiro State Research Supporting Foundation (FAPERJ), and Oswaldo Cruz Foundation (FIOCRUZ).

Conflict of interest

The authors declare no conflicts of interest.

Author details

Mariana Conceição Souza[1,2] and Elaine Cruz Rosas[1,2]*

1 Laboratory of Applied Pharmacology, Farmanguinhos, Oswaldo Cruz Foundation, Rio de Janeiro, Brazil

2 National Institute of Science and Technology of Innovation on Diseases of Neglected Populations (INCT-IDPN), Rio de Janeiro, Brazil

*Address all correspondence to: elaine.rosas@fiocruz.br

References

[1] Soehnlein O, Steffens S, Hidalgo A, Weber C. Neutrophils as protagonists and targets in chronic inflammation. Nature Reviews. Immunology. 2017;**17**(4):248-261

[2] Salzet M, Breton C, Bisogno T, Di Marzo V. Comparative biology of the endocannabinoid system possible role in the immune response. European Journal of Biochemistry. 2000;**267**(16):4917-4927

[3] Berdyshev EV. Cannabinoid receptors and the regulation of immune response. Chemistry and Physics of Lipids. 2000;**108**(1-2):169-190

[4] Pertwee RG. Pharmacological actions of cannabinoids. Handbook of Experimental Pharmacology. 2005;**168**:1-51

[5] Howlett AC, Barth F, Bonner TI, Cabral G, Casellas P, Devane WA, et al. International Union of Pharmacology. XXVII. Classification of cannabinoid receptors. Pharmacological Reviews. 2002;**54**(2):161-202

[6] Fine PG, Rosenfeld MJ. The endocannabinoid system, cannabinoids, and pain. Rambam Maimonides Medical Journal. 2013;**4**(4):e0022

[7] Chakravarti B, Ravi J, Ganju RK. Cannabinoids as therapeutic agents in cancer: Current status and future implications. Oncotarget. 2014;**5**(15):5852-5872

[8] Rossi S, Bernardi G, Centonze D. The endocannabinoid system in the inflammatory and neurodegenerative processes of multiple sclerosis and of amyotrophic lateral sclerosis. Experimental Neurology. 2010;**224**(1):92-102

[9] Immenschuh S. Endocannabinoid signalling as an anti-inflammatory therapeutic target in atherosclerosis: Does it work? Cardiovascular Research. 2009;**84**:341-342

[10] Fukuda S, Kohsaka H, Takayasu A, Yokoyama W, Miyabe C, Miyabe Y, et al. Cannabinoid receptor 2 as a potential therapeutic target in rheumatoid arthritis. BMC Musculoskeletal Disorders. 2014;**15**:275

[11] Lehmann C, Kianian M, Zhou J, Kuster I, Kuschnereit R, Whynot S, et al. Cannabinoid receptor 2 activation reduces intestinal leukocyte recruitment and systemic inflammatory mediator release in acute experimental sepsis. Critical Care. 2012;**16**(2):R47

[12] Schwartz RH, Beveridge RA. Marijuana as an antiemetic drug: How useful is it today? Opinions from clinical oncologists. Journal of Addictive Diseases. 1994;**13**(1):53-65

[13] Mimura T, Oka S, Koshimoto H, Ueda Y, Watanabe Y, Sugiura T. Involvement of the endogenous cannabinoid 2 ligand 2-arachidonyl glycerol in allergic inflammation. International Archives of Allergy and Immunology. 2012;**159**(2):149-156

[14] Lambert DM, Fowler CJ. The endocannabinoid system: Drug targets, lead compounds, and potential therapeutic applications. Journal of Medicinal Chemistry. 2005;**48**(16):5059-5087

[15] Devane WA, Hanus L, Breuer A, Pertwee RG, Stevenson LA, Griffin G, et al. Isolation and structure of a brain constituent that binds to the cannabinoid receptor. Science. 1992;**258**(5090):1946-1949

[16] Mechoulam R, Ben-Shabat S, Hanus L, Ligumsky M, Kaminski NE, Schatz AR, et al. Identification of an endogenous 2-monoglyceride, present

in canine gut, that binds to cannabinoid receptors. Biochemical Pharmacology. 1995;**50**(1):83-90

[17] Sugiura T, Kondo S, Sukagawa A, Nakane S, Shinoda A, Itoh K, et al. 2-Arachidonoylglycerol: A possible endogenous cannabinoid receptor ligand in brain. Biochemical and Biophysical Research Communications. 1995;**215**(1):89-97

[18] Bisogno T, Ligresti A, Di Marzo V. The endocannabinoid signalling system: Biochemical aspects. Pharmacology, Biochemistry, and Behavior. 2005;**81**(2):224-238

[19] Turcotte C, Blanchet MR, Laviolette M, Flamand N. The CB2 receptor and its role as a regulator of inflammation. Cellular and Molecular Life Sciences. 2016;**73**(23):4449-4470

[20] Di Iorio G, Lupi M, Sarchione F, Matarazzo I, Santacroce R, Petruccelli F, et al. The endocannabinoid system: A putative role in neurodegenerative diseases. International Journal of High Risk Behaviors and Addiction. 2013;**2**(3):100-106

[21] Izzo AA, Borrelli F, Capasso R, Di Marzo V, Mechoulam R. Non-psychotropic plant cannabinoids: New therapeutic opportunities from an ancient herb. Trends in Pharmacological Sciences. 2009;**30**(10):515-527

[22] Pertwee RG. The diverse CB1 and CB2 receptor pharmacology of three plant cannabinoids: delta9-tetrahydrocannabinol, cannabidiol, and delta9-tetrahydrocannabivarin. British Journal of Pharmacology. 2008;**153**(2):199-215

[23] Veiga Junior VF, Rosas EC, Carvalho MV, Henriques MG, Pinto AC. Chemical composition and anti-inflammatory activity of copaiba oils from Copaifera cearensis Huber ex Ducke, Copaifera reticulata Ducke and Copaifera multijuga Hayne—A comparative study. Journal of Ethnopharmacology. 2007;**112**(2):248-254

[24] Gertsch J, Pertwee RG, Di Marzo V. Phytocannabinoids beyond the cannabis plant—Do they exist? British Journal of Pharmacology. 2010;**160**(3):523-529

[25] Sharma C, Sadek B, Goyal SN, Sinha S, Kamal MA, Ojha S. Small molecules from nature targeting G-protein coupled cannabinoid receptors: Potential leads for drug discovery and development. Evidence-based Complementary and Alternative Medicine. 2015;**2015**:238482

[26] Gertsch J, Leonti M, Raduner S, Racz I, Chen JZ, Xie XQ, et al. Beta-caryophyllene is a dietary cannabinoid. Proceedings of the National Academy of Sciences of the United States of America. 2008;**105**(26):9099-9104

[27] Gertsch J. Immunomodulatory lipids in plants: Plant fatty acid amides and the human endocannabinoid system. Planta Medica. 2008;**74**(6):638-650

[28] Han S, Thatte J, Buzard DJ, Jones RM. Therapeutic utility of cannabinoid receptor type 2 (CB(2)) selective agonists. Journal of Medicinal Chemistry. 2013;**56**(21):8224-8256

[29] Di Marzo V. New approaches and challenges to targeting the endocannabinoid system. Nature Reviews. Drug Discovery. 2018;**17**(9):623-639

[30] Howlett AC. Cannabinoid receptor signaling. Handbook of Experimental Pharmacology. 2005;**168**:53-79

[31] Bosier B, Muccioli GG, Hermans E, Lambert DM. Functionally selective cannabinoid receptor signalling: Therapeutic implications and opportunities. Biochemical Pharmacology. 2010;**80**(1):1-12

[32] Dhopeshwarkar A, Mackie K. CB2 cannabinoid receptors as a therapeutic target—What does the future hold? Molecular Pharmacology. 2014;**86**(4):430-437

[33] Correa F, Docagne F, Mestre L, Clemente D, Hernangomez M, Loria F, et al. A role for CB2 receptors in anandamide signalling pathways involved in the regulation of IL-12 and IL-23 in microglial cells. Biochemical Pharmacology. 2009;**77**(1):86-100

[34] Correa F, Mestre L, Docagne F, Guaza C. Activation of cannabinoid CB2 receptor negatively regulates IL-12p40 production in murine macrophages: Role of IL-10 and ERK1/2 kinase signaling. British Journal of Pharmacology. 2005;**145**(4):441-448

[35] Correa F, Hernangomez M, Mestre L, Loria F, Spagnolo A, Docagne F, et al. Anandamide enhances IL-10 production in activated microglia by targeting CB(2) receptors: Roles of ERK1/2, JNK, and NF-kappaB. Glia. 2010;**58**(2):135-147

[36] Rajesh M, Mukhopadhyay P, Hasko G, Huffman JW, Mackie K, Pacher P. CB2 cannabinoid receptor agonists attenuate TNF-alpha-induced human vascular smooth muscle cell proliferation and migration. British Journal of Pharmacology. 2008;**153**(2):347-357

[37] Borner C, Smida M, Hollt V, Schraven B, Kraus J. Cannabinoid receptor type 1- and 2-mediated increase in cyclic AMP inhibits T cell receptor-triggered signaling. The Journal of Biological Chemistry. 2009;**284**(51):35450-35460

[38] Howlett AC, Shim JY. Cannabinoid Receptors and Signal Transduction. In: Madame Curie Bioscience Database [Internet]. Austin (TX): Landes Bioscience; 2000-2013. Available from: https://www.ncbi.nlm.nih.gov/books/NBK6154/

[39] Fride E, Foox A, Rosenberg E, Faigenboim M, Cohen V, Barda L, et al. Milk intake and survival in newborn cannabinoid CB1 receptor knockout mice: Evidence for a "CB3" receptor. European Journal of Pharmacology. 2003;**461**(1):27-34

[40] Irving A, Abdulrazzaq G, Chan SLF, Penman J, Harvey J, Alexander SPH. Cannabinoid receptor-related orphan G protein-coupled receptors. Advances in Pharmacology. 2017;**80**:223-247

[41] Liu J, Li H, Burstein SH, Zurier RB, Chen JD. Activation and binding of peroxisome proliferator-activated receptor gamma by synthetic cannabinoid ajulemic acid. Molecular Pharmacology. 2003;**63**(5):983-992

[42] Ambrosio AL, Dias SM, Polikarpov I, Zurier RB, Burstein SH, Garratt RC. Ajulemic acid, a synthetic nonpsychoactive cannabinoid acid, bound to the ligand binding domain of the human peroxisome proliferator-activated receptor gamma. The Journal of Biological Chemistry. 2007;**282**(25):18625-18633

[43] O'Sullivan SE. Cannabinoids go nuclear: Evidence for activation of peroxisome proliferator-activated receptors. British Journal of Pharmacology. 2007;**152**(5):576-582

[44] Abood ME, Martin BR. Neurobiology of marijuana abuse. Trends in Pharmacological Sciences. 1992;**13**(5):201-206

[45] Marsicano G, Lutz B. Expression of the cannabinoid receptor CB1 in distinct neuronal subpopulations in the adult mouse forebrain. The European Journal of Neuroscience. 1999;**11**(12):4213-4225

[46] Devane WA, Dysarz FA 3rd, Johnson MR, Melvin LS, Howlett AC. Determination and characterization of a cannabinoid receptor in rat

brain. Molecular Pharmacology. 1988;**34**(5):605-613

[47] Hernandez-Cervantes R, Mendez-Diaz M, Prospero-Garcia O, Morales-Montor J. Immunoregulatory role of cannabinoids during infectious disease. Neuroimmunomodulation. 2017;**24**(4-5):183-199

[48] Deng L, Guindon J, Cornett BL, Makriyannis A, Mackie K, Hohmann AG. Chronic cannabinoid receptor 2 activation reverses paclitaxel neuropathy without tolerance or cannabinoid receptor 1-dependent withdrawal. Biological Psychiatry. 2015;**77**(5):475-487

[49] Navarro G, Morales P, Rodriguez-Cueto C, Fernandez-Ruiz J, Jagerovic N, Franco R. Targeting cannabinoid CB2 receptors in the central nervous system. Medicinal chemistry approaches with focus on neurodegenerative disorders. Frontiers in Neuroscience. 2016;**10**:406

[50] Bouaboula M, Rinaldi M, Carayon P, Carillon C, Delpech B, Shire D, et al. Cannabinoid-receptor expression in human leukocytes. European Journal of Biochemistry. 1993;**214**(1):173-180

[51] Galiegue S, Mary S, Marchand J, Dussossoy D, Carriere D, Carayon P, et al. Expression of central and peripheral cannabinoid receptors in human immune tissues and leukocyte subpopulations. European Journal of Biochemistry. 1995;**232**(1):54-61

[52] Carlisle SJ, Marciano-Cabral F, Staab A, Ludwick C, Cabral GA. Differential expression of the CB2 cannabinoid receptor by rodent macrophages and macrophage-like cells in relation to cell activation. International Immunopharmacology. 2002;**2**(1):69-82

[53] Klein TW. Cannabinoid-based drugs as anti-inflammatory therapeutics. Nature Reviews. Immunology. 2005;**5**(5):400-411

[54] Bento AF, Marcon R, Dutra RC, Claudino RF, Cola M, Leite DF, et al. Beta-caryophyllene inhibits dextran sulfate sodium-induced colitis in mice through CB2 receptor activation and PPARgamma pathway. The American Journal of Pathology. 2011;**178**(3):1153-1166

[55] Singh UP, Singh NP, Singh B, Price RL, Nagarkatti M, Nagarkatti PS. Cannabinoid receptor-2 (CB2) agonist ameliorates colitis in IL-10(−/−) mice by attenuating the activation of T cells and promoting their apoptosis. Toxicology and Applied Pharmacology. 2012;**258**(2):256-267

[56] Murikinati S, Juttler E, Keinert T, Ridder DA, Muhammad S, Waibler Z, et al. Activation of cannabinoid 2 receptors protects against cerebral ischemia by inhibiting neutrophil recruitment. The FASEB Journal. 2010;**24**(3):788-798

[57] Tschop J, Kasten KR, Nogueiras R, Goetzman HS, Cave CM, England LG, et al. The cannabinoid receptor 2 is critical for the host response to sepsis. Journal of Immunology. 2009;**183**(1):499-505

[58] Toguri JT, Lehmann C, Laprairie RB, Szczesniak AM, Zhou J, Denovan-Wright EM, et al. Anti-inflammatory effects of cannabinoid CB(2) receptor activation in endotoxin-induced uveitis. British Journal of Pharmacology. 2014;**171**(6):1448-1461

[59] Smith SR, Denhardt G, Terminelli C. The anti-inflammatory activities of cannabinoid receptor ligands in mouse peritonitis models. European Journal of Pharmacology. 2001;**432**(1):107-119

[60] Semerad CL, Liu F, Gregory AD, Stumpf K, Link DC. G-CSF is an essential regulator of neutrophil trafficking from the bone marrow to the blood. Immunity. 2002;**17**(4):413-423

[61] Sadik CD, Kim ND, Luster AD. Neutrophils cascading their way to inflammation. Trends in Immunology. 2011;**32**(10):452-460

[62] Balenga NA, Aflaki E, Kargl J, Platzer W, Schroder R, Blattermann S, et al. GPR55 regulates cannabinoid 2 receptor-mediated responses in human neutrophils. Cell Research. 2011;**21**(10):1452-1469

[63] Pillinger MH, Abramson SB. The neutrophil in rheumatoid arthritis. Rheumatic Diseases Clinics of North America. 1995;**21**(3):691-714

[64] Springer TA. Traffic signals for lymphocyte recirculation and leukocyte emigration: The multistep paradigm. Cell. 1994;**76**(2):301-314

[65] Bokoch GM. Regulation of innate immunity by rho GTPases. Trends in Cell Biology. 2005;**15**(3):163-171

[66] Graham ES, Angel CE, Schwarcz LE, Dunbar PR, Glass M. Detailed characterisation of CB2 receptor protein expression in peripheral blood immune cells from healthy human volunteers using flow cytometry. International Journal of Immunopathology and Pharmacology. 2010;**23**(1):25-34

[67] Derocq JM, Jbilo O, Bouaboula M, Segui M, Clere C, Casellas P. Genomic and functional changes induced by the activation of the peripheral cannabinoid receptor CB2 in the promyelocytic cells HL-60. Possible involvement of the CB2 receptor in cell differentiation. The Journal of Biological Chemistry. 2000;**275**(21):15621-15628

[68] Alberich Jorda M, Rayman N, Tas M, Verbakel SE, Battista N, van Lom K, et al. The peripheral cannabinoid receptor Cb2, frequently expressed on AML blasts, either induces a neutrophilic differentiation block or confers abnormal migration properties in a ligand-dependent manner. Blood. 2004;**104**(2):526-534

[69] Kurihara R, Tohyama Y, Matsusaka S, Naruse H, Kinoshita E, Tsujioka T, et al. Effects of peripheral cannabinoid receptor ligands on motility and polarization in neutrophil-like HL60 cells and human neutrophils. The Journal of Biological Chemistry. 2006;**281**(18):12908-12918

[70] McHugh D, Tanner C, Mechoulam R, Pertwee RG, Ross RA. Inhibition of human neutrophil chemotaxis by endogenous cannabinoids and phytocannabinoids: Evidence for a site distinct from CB1 and CB2. Molecular Pharmacology. 2008;**73**(2):441-450

[71] Berdyshev E, Boichot E, Corbel M, Germain N, Lagente V. Effects of cannabinoid receptor ligands on LPS-induced pulmonary inflammation in mice. Life Sciences. 1998;**63**(8):Pl125-Pl129

[72] Jorda MA, Rayman N, Valk P, De Wee E, Delwel R. Identification, characterization, and function of a novel oncogene: The peripheral cannabinoid receptor Cb2. Annals of the New York Academy of Sciences. 2003;**996**:10-16

[73] Mukhopadhyay P, Rajesh M, Horvath B, Batkai S, Park O, Tanchian G, et al. Cannabidiol protects against hepatic ischemia/reperfusion injury by attenuating inflammatory signaling and response, oxidative/nitrative stress, and cell death. Free Radical Biology & Medicine. 2011;**50**(10):1368-1381

[74] Wang Y, Mukhopadhyay P, Cao Z, Wang H, Feng D, Hasko G, et al. Cannabidiol attenuates alcohol-induced liver steatosis, metabolic dysregulation, inflammation and neutrophil-mediated injury. Scientific Reports. 2017;7(1):12064

[75] Ribeiro A, Ferraz-de-Paula V, Pinheiro ML, Vitoretti LB, Mariano-Souza DP, Quinteiro-Filho WM, et al. Cannabidiol, a non-psychotropic plant-derived cannabinoid, decreases inflammation in a murine model of acute lung injury: Role for the adenosine A(2A) receptor. European Journal of Pharmacology. 2012;**678**(1-3):78-85

[76] Napimoga MH, Benatti BB, Lima FO, Alves PM, Campos AC, Pena-Dos-Santos DR, et al. Cannabidiol decreases bone resorption by inhibiting RANK/RANKL expression and pro-inflammatory cytokines during experimental periodontitis in rats. International Immunopharmacology. 2009;**9**(2):216-222

[77] Thapa D, Cairns EA, Szczesniak AM, Toguri JT, Caldwell MD, Kelly MEM. The cannabinoids Delta(8) THC, CBD, and HU-308 act via distinct receptors to reduce corneal pain and inflammation. Cannabis and Cannabinoid Research. 2018;**3**(1):11-20

[78] Makwana R, Venkatasamy R, Spina D, Page C. The effect of phytocannabinoids on airway hyper-responsiveness, airway inflammation, and cough. The Journal of Pharmacology and Experimental Therapeutics. 2015;**353**(1):169-180

[79] Li W, Huang H, Niu X, Fan T, Mu Q, Li H. Protective effect of tetrahydrocoptisine against ethanol-induced gastric ulcer in mice. Toxicology and Applied Pharmacology. 2013;**272**(1):21-29

[80] Horvath B, Mukhopadhyay P, Kechrid M, Patel V, Tanchian G, Wink DA, et al. Beta-caryophyllene ameliorates cisplatin-induced nephrotoxicity in a cannabinoid 2 receptor-dependent manner. Free Radical Biology & Medicine. 2012;**52**(8):1325-1333

[81] Medeiros R, Passos GF, Vitor CE, Koepp J, Mazzuco TL, Pianowski LF, et al. Effect of two active compounds obtained from the essential oil of Cordia verbenacea on the acute inflammatory responses elicited by LPS in the rat paw. British Journal of Pharmacology. 2007;**151**(5):618-627

[82] Varga ZV, Matyas C, Erdelyi K, Cinar R, Nieri D, Chicca A, et al. Beta-caryophyllene protects against alcoholic steatohepatitis by attenuating inflammation and metabolic dysregulation in mice. British Journal of Pharmacology. 2018;**175**(2):320-334

[83] Andrade-Silva M, Correa LB, Candea AL, Cavalher-Machado SC, Barbosa HS, Rosas EC, et al. The cannabinoid 2 receptor agonist beta-caryophyllene modulates the inflammatory reaction induced by *Mycobacterium bovis* BCG by inhibiting neutrophil migration. Inflammation Research. 2016;**65**(11):869-879

[84] Montecucco F, Di Marzo V, da Silva RF, Vuilleumier N, Capettini L, Lenglet S, et al. The activation of the cannabinoid receptor type 2 reduces neutrophilic protease-mediated vulnerability in atherosclerotic plaques. European Heart Journal. 2012;**33**(7):846-856

[85] Nilsson O, Fowler CJ, Jacobsson SO. The cannabinoid agonist WIN 55,212-2 inhibits TNF-alpha-induced neutrophil transmigration across ECV304 cells. European Journal of Pharmacology. 2006;**547**(1-3):165-173

[86] Hasenoehrl C, Storr M, Schicho R. Cannabinoids for treating inflammatory bowel diseases: Where are we and where do we go? Expert Review of Gastroenterology & Hepatology. 2017;**11**(4):329-337

[87] Borrelli F, Fasolino I, Romano B, Capasso R, Maiello F, Coppola D, et al. Beneficial effect of the

non-psychotropic plant cannabinoid cannabigerol on experimental inflammatory bowel disease. Biochemical Pharmacology. 2013;**85**(9):1306-1316

[88] Schicho R, Bashashati M, Bawa M, McHugh D, Saur D, Hu HM, et al. The atypical cannabinoid O-1602 protects against experimental colitis and inhibits neutrophil recruitment. Inflammatory Bowel Diseases. 2011;**17**(8):1651-1664

[89] Uranga JA, Vera G, Abalo R. Cannabinoid pharmacology and therapy in gut disorders. Biochemical Pharmacology. 2018;**157**:134-147

[90] Rosas E, Correa L, MdG H. In: Khajah MA, editor. Neutrophils in Rheumatoid Arthritis: A Target for Discovering New Therapies Based on Natural Products. 1st ed. Rijeka, Croatia: IntechOpen; 2017. pp. 89-118

[91] Richardson D, Pearson RG, Kurian N, Latif ML, Garle MJ, Barrett DA, et al. Characterisation of the cannabinoid receptor system in synovial tissue and fluid in patients with osteoarthritis and rheumatoid arthritis. Arthritis Research & Therapy. 2008;**10**(2):R43

[92] Gui H, Liu X, Wang ZW, He DY, Su DF, Dai SM. Expression of cannabinoid receptor 2 and its inhibitory effects on synovial fibroblasts in rheumatoid arthritis. Rheumatology (Oxford, England). 2014;**53**(5):802-809

[93] Duerr GD, Heinemann JC, Gestrich C, Heuft T, Klaas T, Keppel K, et al. Impaired border zone formation and adverse remodeling after reperfused myocardial infarction in cannabinoid CB2 receptor deficient mice. Life Sciences. 2015;**138**:8-17

[94] Kobayashi SD, Voyich JM, DeLeo FR. Regulation of the neutrophil-mediated inflammatory response to infection. Microbes and Infection. 2003;**5**(14):1337-1344

[95] Linken A. A study of drug-taking among young patients attending a clinic for venereal diseases. The British Journal of Venereal Diseases. 1968;**44**(4):337-341

[96] Smith D, Rose AJ. Observations in the Haight-Ashbury Medical Clinic of San Francisco. Health problems in a "hippie" subculture. Clinical Pediatrics (Phila). 1968;**7**(6):313-316

[97] Sonego F, Castanheira FV, Ferreira RG, Kanashiro A, Leite CA, Nascimento DC, et al. Paradoxical roles of the neutrophil in sepsis: Protective and deleterious. Frontiers in Immunology. 2016;**7**:155

[98] Zhang H, Sun B. Pleiotropic regulations of neutrophil receptors response to sepsis. Inflammation Research. 2017;**66**(3):197-207

[99] Shen XF, Cao K, Jiang JP, Guan WX, Du JF. Neutrophil dysregulation during sepsis: An overview and update. Journal of Cellular and Molecular Medicine. 2017;**21**(9):1687-1697

[100] Kapellos TS, Recio C, Greaves DR, Iqbal AJ. Cannabinoid receptor 2 modulates neutrophil recruitment in a murine model of endotoxemia. Mediators of Inflammation. 2017;**2017**:4315412

[101] Leite-Avalca MC, Lomba LA, Bastos-Pereira AL, Brito HO, Fraga D, Zampronio AR. Involvement of central endothelin ETA and cannabinoid CB1 receptors and arginine vasopressin release in sepsis induced by cecal ligation and puncture in rats. Shock. 2016;**46**(3):290-296

[102] Kianian M, Kelly ME, Zhou J, Hung O, Cerny V, Rowden G, et al. Cannabinoid receptor 1 inhibition improves the intestinal microcirculation in experimental endotoxemia. Clinical Hemorheology and Microcirculation. 2014;**58**(2):333-342

[103] Kadoi Y, Hinohara H, Kunimoto F, Kuwano H, Saito S, Goto F. Effects of AM281, a cannabinoid antagonist, on systemic haemodynamics, internal carotid artery blood flow and mortality in septic shock in rats. British Journal of Anaesthesia. 2005;**94**(5):563-568

[104] Kadoi Y, Goto F. Effects of AM281, a cannabinoid antagonist, on circulatory deterioration and cytokine production in an endotoxin shock model: Comparison with norepinephrine. Journal of Anesthesia. 2006;**20**(4):284-289

[105] Kaufmann SHE, Dorhoi A, Hotchkiss RS, Bartenschlager R. Host-directed therapies for bacterial and viral infections. Nature Reviews. Drug Discovery. 2018;**17**(1):35-56

Chapter 3

Neutrophil Activation by Antibody Receptors

Carlos Rosales and Eileen Uribe-Querol

Abstract

Neutrophils, the most abundant leukocytes in blood, are relevant cells of both the innate and the adaptive immune system. Immunoglobulin (Ig) G antibody molecules are crucial activators of neutrophils. IgGs identify many types of pathogens via their two Fab portions and are in turn detected through their Fc portion by specific Fcγ receptors (FcγRs) on the membrane of neutrophils. Thus, antibodies bring the specificity of the adaptive immune response to the potent antimicrobial and inflammatory functions of neutrophils. Two types of FcγRs with several polymorphic variants exist on the human neutrophil. These receptors are considered to be redundant in inducing cell responses. Yet, new evidence presented in recent years on how the particular IgG subclass and the glycosylation pattern of the antibody modulate the IgG–FcγR interaction has suggested that a particular effector function may in fact be activated in response to a specific type of FcγR. In this chapter, we describe the main types of FcγRs on neutrophils and our current view on how particular FcγRs activate various signaling pathways to promote unique effector cell functions, including phagocytosis, activation of integrins, nuclear factor activation, and formation of neutrophil extracellular traps (NETs).

Keywords: neutrophil, phagocytosis, degranulation, NETs, antibody, Fc receptors, integrins, NF-κB

1. Introduction

Neutrophils are the most abundant cell type in human blood. They are produced in the bone marrow and then released into the circulation. At sites of infection or inflammation, neutrophils migrate to tissues, where they complete their functions. Finally, neutrophils die by apoptosis and are eliminated by macrophages. Neutrophils are an essential part of the innate immune system [1], with significant antimicrobial functions, including phagocytosis, degranulation, and the formation of neutrophil extracellular traps (NETs). These antimicrobial functions were believed to be the only goal of neutrophils. However, it has recently become clear that neutrophils display many functional responses that go beyond the simple killing of microorganisms. Neutrophils produce cytokines [2] and other inflammatory factors [3] that regulate the whole immune system [4, 5]. Consequently, neutrophils are also key effector cells of the adaptive immune system.

Immunoglobulin (Ig) G antibody molecules are an essential part of the adaptive immune system. IgGs recognize antigens via their two Fab portions and are in turn linked through their Fc portion to specific Fcγ receptors (FcγRs) on the membrane of leukocytes [6, 7]. In this way, antibodies function as a bridge between the specific adaptive immune response and the potent innate immune functions of leukocytes. In the human neutrophil, two types of FcγR exist. Thus, antibodies are important activators of neutrophils. The Fcγ receptors on the neutrophil are considered to be redundant in inducing cell responses [8, 9]. However, recent findings on how a particular IgG subclass and the glycosylation pattern of the antibody regulate the IgG–FcγR interaction suggest that a particular effector function may in fact be activated in response to a specific type of FcγR. It is the purpose of this chapter to describe the FcγRs on human neutrophils and present our current view of how particular FcγRs activate various signaling pathways to promote unique effector cell functions.

2. Neutrophils

Neutrophils are the most abundant leukocytes in blood and because they are the first cells to appear at sites of inflammation and infection; they are regarded as the first line of defense of the innate immune system [10]. Neutrophils can rapidly move from the blood into affected sites through a process known as the leukocyte adhesion cascade. Once in the tissues, they perform important antimicrobial functions, including phagocytosis, degranulation, and formation of neutrophil extracellular traps (NETs) [11, 12].

2.1 Leukocyte adhesion cascade

Neutrophils leave the blood circulation at sites of infection or inflammation by binding to the endothelial cells and then transmigrating into the tissues [13]. This process known, as the leukocyte adhesion cascade (**Figure 1**), begins with the activation of endothelial cells at the affected site. Activated endothelial cells upregulate the expression of adhesion receptors such as E- and P-selectins. Neutrophils bind to these selectins via glycoprotein ligands on their membrane. As a consequence, neutrophils can then roll on endothelial cells. Next, neutrophils get activated by chemokines, which induce a high affinity state on integrins, another group of adhesion receptors. Binding of integrins with their corresponding ligands, such as intercellular adhesion molecule-1 (ICAM-1) and ICAM-2 on endothelial cells, results in slower neutrophil rolling and then firm adhesion that makes neutrophils stop. Finally, neutrophils transmigrate the endothelium into the tissues. Engagement of endothelial-cell adhesion molecules seems to provoke the opening of endothelial-cell contacts by redistributing junctional molecules in a way that promotes transmigration of neutrophils. Molecules that do not help neutrophil migration, such as vascular endothelial cadherin (VE-cadherin), are moved away from junctional regions. Other endothelial junctional molecules for which neutrophils express ligands concentrate on the endothelial cell luminal surface creating an adhesive environment for the neutrophil. Platelet/endothelial-cell adhesion molecule 1 (PECAM1) and CD99 support homophilic interactions between endothelial cells and neutrophils. While, junctional adhesion molecule (JAM)-1 and JAM-2 on the endothelial cell bind to the β1 integrin VLA4, and the β2 integrins LFA-1 and Mac-1 on the neutrophil, respectively. The endothelial cell-selective adhesion molecule (ESAM) is also involved in transmigration by binding to an unknown

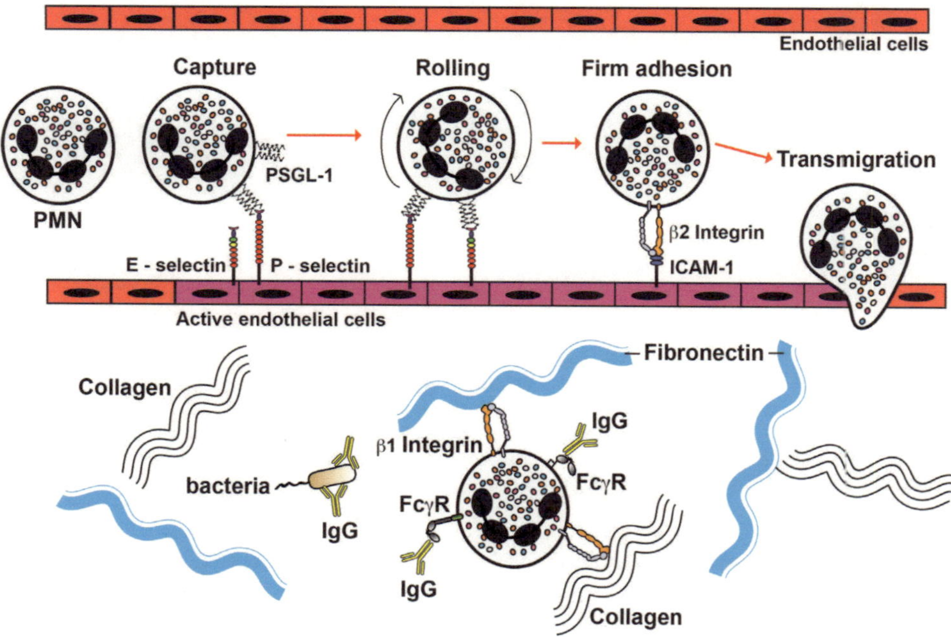

Figure 1.
Leukocyte adhesion cascade. Neutrophils, also known as polymorphonuclear (PMN) cells, move to sites of inflammation via a leukocyte adhesion cascade that includes activation of endothelial cells with upregulation of E- and P-selectins. Neutrophils bind to these selectins via glycoprotein ligands, such as P-selectin glycoprotein ligand-1 (PSGL-1), and begin rolling on endothelial cells. Next, neutrophils get stimulated by chemokines and activate their β2 integrins, which bind to their corresponding ligands, such as intercellular adhesion molecule-1 (ICAM-1). Integrin binding induces firm adhesion and transmigration of neutrophils into tissues. Once in tissues, neutrophils move following chemoattractant gradients to reach affected sites using now adhesion of β1 integrins to proteins of the extracellular matrix, such as collagen and fibronectin. Antibodies (IgG) bind to microorganisms (bacteria) and are in turn recognized by Fcγ receptors (FcγR) on the membrane of neutrophils.

ligand on neutrophils [12, 14]. Once neutrophils move into tissues, they follow chemoattractant gradients to reach affected sites using now adhesion of β1 integrins to proteins of the extracellular matrix, such as collagen and fibronectin [15] (**Figure 1**). Important chemoattractants for neutrophils are activated complement components, such as the anaphylatoxin C5a, bacterial components, such as formyl-methionyl-leucyl-phenylalanine (fMLF) and cytokines, such as interleukin (IL) 8.

2.2 Antimicrobial mechanisms of neutrophils

Neutrophils recruited from the circulation into infected tissues can eliminate microorganisms by phagocytosis, by releasing antimicrobial substances or by forming NETs [11, 12] (**Figure 2**).

2.2.1 Phagocytosis

Phagocytosis is the process by which particles larger than 5 μm get internalized by the cell into a vacuole called the phagosome. Neutrophils recognize pathogens directly through pattern-recognition receptors (PAMPs), or indirectly through opsonin receptors. Opsonins are host proteins, such as antibody molecules or complement components, that bind to microorganisms and facilitate their detection and destruction by leukocytes [16, 17]. After internalization, the nascent phagosome matures by fusing with lysosomes [18]. During maturation, antimicrobial

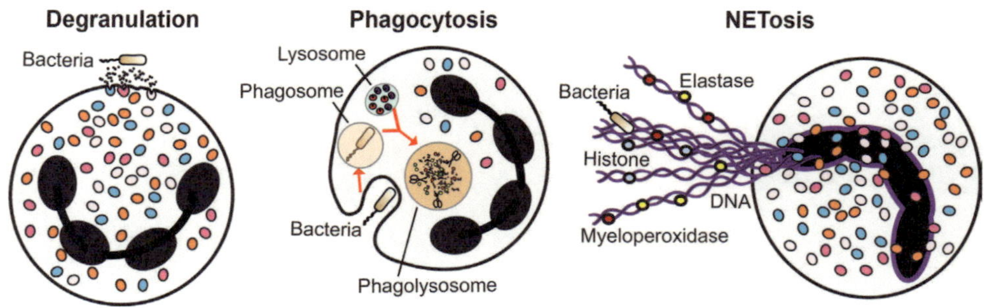

Figure 2.
Antimicrobial mechanisms of neutrophils. Neutrophils can destroy microbial pathogens, such as bacteria by (a) degranulation, (b) phagocytosis, and (c) NETosis. During degranulation, antimicrobial proteins are released outside the neutrophil. In phagocytosis, the pathogen is ingested in a vacuole named phagosome, which then fuses to lysosomes and becomes a phagolysosome, where the pathogen is destroyed. During NETosis, DNA fibers decorated with histones and granular proteins, such as elastase and myeloperoxidase are released in structures known as neutrophil extracellular traps (NETs).

molecules are delivered into the phagosomal lumen, and the vesicle is transformed into a phagolysosome [19]. In the phagolysosome, reactive oxygen species (ROS) are produced by the NADPH oxidase on the phagosomal membrane, and the pH inside drops to 4.5–5. Also, hydrogen peroxide (H_2O_2) is converted to hypochlorous acid (HOCl) in a reaction catalyzed by myeloperoxidase (MPO) [20]. Together, these actions form a toxic environment for the microorganism.

2.2.2 Degranulation

During neutrophil formation in the bone marrow, immature neutrophils synthesize proteins that are sorted into different granules [10]. Granules are classified into three different types based on their content. Azurophilic granules contain mainly myeloperoxidase, elastase, and cathepsin G. Specific granules contain mainly collagenase, lactoferrin, and lysozyme. Gelatinase granules contain mainly gelatinase, lysozyme, and cytochrome b558 [21]. Neutrophils also form secretory vesicles at the last step of their differentiation. These secretory vesicles contain several important receptors on their membrane, including complement receptors (CR1), Fc receptors (CD16), lipopolysaccharide (LPS) receptors (CD-14), and fMLF receptors. Granule heterogeneity is due to the controlled expression of the granule protein genes [22]. Mature neutrophils are released into the circulation and when they reach sites of infection, neutrophils can degranulate in order to deliver their antimicrobial proteins. Secretory vesicles present the greatest predisposition for extracellular release, followed by gelatinase granules, specific granules, and azurophil granules [23]. The hierarchical mobilization of neutrophil granules and secretory vesicles depend on intracellular Ca^{2+}-level [24].

2.2.3 Neutrophil extracellular traps (NETs)

When neutrophils cannot ingest large microorganisms, they can display another antimicrobial strategy [25]. Neutrophils can release long chromatin fibers that are decorated with proteins from their granules. These fibers can trap microorganisms, and therefore, they have been called neutrophil extracellular traps (NETs) [26]. The process of NETs formation is called NETosis [27]. NETosis has been described as a special form of programmed cell death. The complete mechanisms of NETs formation are still unknown; it seems that NETosis requires NADPH oxidase activation, reactive oxygen species (ROS) production, myeloperoxidase (MPO), and neutrophil elastase (NE) release [28, 29] (**Figure 2**).

3. Fcγ receptors

Antibodies produced by the adaptive immune response are mainly of the IgG class. These antibodies present higher affinity and greater specificity for their particular antigen. Thus, IgG antibodies are key for controlling infections from all types of pathogens, including viruses, bacteria, fungi, and protozoa [30]. However, IgG molecules do not directly damage the microorganisms they recognize. It is in fact, the cells of the innate immune system, which are responsible for the antimicrobial functions of these antibodies. Although, some antibodies can activate complement, which is then deposited on microorganisms to promote phagocytosis via complement receptors [17, 31], or to induce bacterial lysis via the formation of the membrane attack complex [32], most IgG antibodies bind to specific receptors on the membrane of leukocytes [7, 8]. These receptors recognize the fragment crystallizable (Fc) portion of IgG molecules and are therefore known as Fcγ receptors (FcγR). Cross-linking of FcγR on the surface of cells activates several antimicrobial functions [6].

3.1 Human Fcγ receptors

Human Fcγ receptors comprise a family of glycoproteins expressed on the membrane of immune cells [7, 8]. These receptors can bind to the various IgG subclasses with different affinities [7], and induce different cellular responses [6]. FcγR can be classified as activating receptors (FcγRI/CD64, FcγRIIa/CD32a, FcγRIIIa/CD16a, and FcγRIIIb/CD16b), and one inhibitory receptor (FcγRIIb/CD32b) [7, 9, 33, 34] (**Figure 3**).

FcγRI is a high affinity receptor, having three Ig-like extracellular domains. It binds mainly monomeric IgG [9]. In contrast, FcγRII and FcγRIII are low-affinity receptors, having two Ig-like extracellular domains. They bind only multimeric immune complexes [9, 35]. FcγRI is associated with a dimer of the common Fc receptor γ chain, which contains an immunoreceptor tyrosine-based activation motif (ITAM) sequence (**Figure 3**). The ITAM sequence is important for receptor signaling [36].

FcγRIIa contains its own ITAM within its cytoplasmic tail. In contrast, the inhibitory receptor FcγRIIb contains an immunoreceptor tyrosine-based inhibition

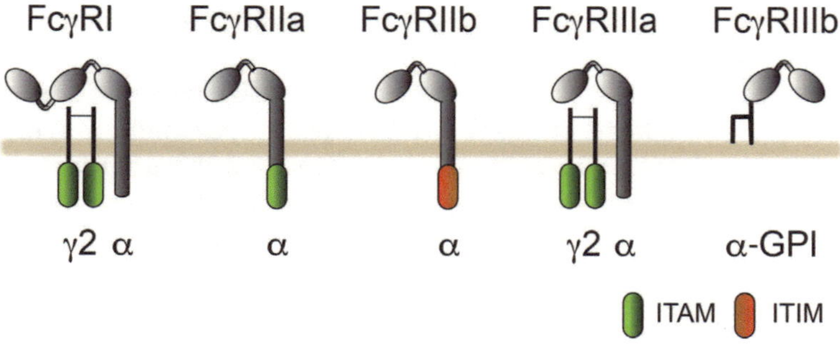

Figure 3.
Human Fcγ receptors. Schematic illustration of human receptors for IgG. Fcγ receptors are shown relative to the cell membrane (brown line). The IgG-binding chain (α) is expressed together with their respective γ2 signaling subunits. FcγRI is a high affinity receptor, having three Ig-like extracellular domains. FcγRII and FcγRIII are low-affinity receptors, having two Ig-like extracellular domains. FcγRIIIb is expressed exclusively on neutrophils, and it is a glycosylphosphatidylinositol (GPI)-linked receptor missing a cytoplasmic tail. ITAM, immunoreceptor tyrosine-based activation motif with consensus sequence YxxI/Lx $_{(6–12)}$YxxI/L [36] (green oval); ITIM, immunoreceptor tyrosine-based inhibitory motif with the consensus sequence I/V/L/SxYxxL/V [39] (red oval).

motif (ITIM) within its cytoplasmic tail (**Figure 3**). The FcγRIIb negatively regulates various cell functions including antibody production by the B cell [37], proliferation, degranulation, and phagocytosis in other leukocytes when it is cross-linked with activating FcγRs [38, 39]. Most leukocytes express both activating and inhibitory FcγRs, hence simultaneous cross-linking establishes a threshold for cell activation [40] that maintains a balanced immune response [41, 42].

FcγRIII has two isoforms: FcγRIIIa is a receptor with a transmembrane domain and a cytoplasmic tail, associated with an ITAM-containing homodimer of Fc receptor γ chains (**Figure 3**). It is expressed mainly on macrophages, natural killer (NK) cells, and dendritic cells [7, 8]. In contrast, FcγRIIIb is expressed exclusively on neutrophils and it is a glycosylphosphatidylinositol (GPI)-linked receptor missing a cytoplasmic tail. Also, no other subunits are known to associate with it (**Figure 3**). It is important to mention that human FcγRIIa and FcγRIIIb are exclusive receptors that are not found in other species [33, 43].

4. IgG binding to Fcγ receptors

As mentioned before, there is one high-affinity Fcγ receptor, FcγRI (CD64), and two groups of low-affinity Fcγ receptors, FcγRII and FcγRIII (**Figure 3**). This causes that a single IgG molecule cannot bind to most Fcγ receptors. However, when IgG molecules form antigen-antibody (immune) complexes, they can have many low affinity interactions with Fcγ receptors. Thus, only immune complexes are able to induce the cross-linking of FcγR required for the activation of various antibody-mediated cell functions. It is clear then that depending on the nature of the immune complex, the interaction with various FcγR will change. Several factors have been identified as having an important influence on the affinity of antibody molecules for particular FcγRs. These factors include the type of IgG subclass [7, 44], the IgG glycosylation pattern [45, 46], and receptor polymorphisms.

4.1 The type of IgG subclass

There are four subclasses of IgG (IgG1, IgG2a, IgG2b, and IgG3 in mice; and IgG1, IgG2, IgG3, and IgG4 in humans) [47]. This leads to the formation of different types of immune complexes. Several *in vivo* studies have indeed suggested that different IgG subclasses can activate particular cell responses. For example, in mice, IgG2b was better than IgG1 at eliminating B cell [48] and T cell lymphomas [49]. Also, antierythrocyte antibodies of IgG2a and IgG2b subclasses were better than antibodies of IgG1 and IgG3 subclasses in mediating phagocytosis of opsonized erythrocytes [50]. In humans, it was shown that most FcγRs bind primarily IgG1 and IgG3 over the other subclasses of IgG [6, 7]. Together, these reports confirm that different IgG subclasses mediate different cellular responses *in vivo,* and suggest that different cellular activities result from cross-linking different FcγRs. However, the mechanism used to generate this IgG-FcγR selectivity is not completely understood. Accordingly, a great interest exists for determining which type of IgG binds to which FcγR and what particular receptor is involved in mediating a certain cellular function.

Obviously, this selectivity depends mainly on the affinities of different IgG subclasses to particular Fcγ receptors. For this reason, detailed studies to measure the affinities of IgG subclasses to the various Fcγ receptors have been conducted both for mice FcγRs [51] and for all human FcγRs [35]. Through these studies, it was found that IgG1 and IgG3 bind to all FcγR. IgG2 binds mainly to FcγRIIa (H_{131} isoform), and FcγRIIIa (V_{158} isoform), but not to FcγRIIIb [35]. IgG4 binds to many FcγRs [35]. Thus, it is clear that different IgG subclasses engage different Fcγ receptors depending on the relative affinity of these receptors for a particular IgG class [33].

4.2 The IgG glycosylation pattern

All IgG molecules are glycoproteins with an N-glycosylated carbohydrate side chain that is important for antibody function [52]. Deletion of this carbohydrate (sugar) side chain results in poor binding to FcγRs [53]. The N-glycans are heterogeneous in their sugar composition and are attached to asparagine 297 (Asp^{297}) in the Fc portion of the IgG [54]. The carbohydrate side chain may contain sugar residues such as galactose, fucose, and sialic acid in straight or branching patterns [46], and the differences in the glycosylation pattern seem to regulate IgG activity [55].

Many IgG antibodies present a fucose residue linked to an N-acetylglucosamine residue [56]. When this residue is removed, IgG molecules present an increased affinity to the FcγRIIIa [57], and also an increase in antibody-dependent cell cytotoxicity (ADCC) activity against various tumor cells [51, 57, 58]. Based on these findings, recombinant IgG antibodies with low fucose levels have been produced in order to increase their ADCC activity. Several of these antibodies are now in clinical trials to test their therapeutic potential [59].

Many IgG antibodies also present a carbohydrate side chain that terminates with sialic acid residues [60]. Contrary to antibodies without fucose, terminal sialic acid usually correlates with low affinity for FcγRs and also with lower ADCC activity [61, 62]. Interestingly, these sialic acid-rich antibodies seem to preferentially bind other receptors different from FcγRs. The receptor dendritic cell specific ICAM-3 grabbing nonintegrin (DC-SIGN) was identified as a receptor for sialic acid-rich IgG [63]. Therefore, terminal sialic acid can modify IgG activity by promoting less binding to FcγRs and more binding to other receptors [45].

4.3 Polymorphisms of receptors

Another factor influencing the affinity of antibody molecules is the existence of several polymorphisms for the unique FcγRIIa and FcγRIIIb present on human neutrophils [64]. There are two isoforms for FcγRIIa with different amino acids at position 131. These are identified as low-responder (H_{131}) and high-responder (R_{131}) [65]. Similarly, for FcγRIIIb two isoforms exist differing at four positions, NA1 (R36 N65 D82 V106) and NA2 (S36 S65 N82 I106) [66], and with different glycosylation patterns [67]. In addition, another FcγRIIIb isoform named SH is generated by a point mutation (A78D) in the NA2 allele [68]. These multiple FcγR isoforms display diverse binding affinity for different IgG classes [35], creating variable cell responses to different antibodies.

5. Fcγ receptor signaling

The human neutrophil expresses two unique activating Fc receptors: FcγRIIa and FcγRIIIb. FcγRIIa is a receptor containing ITAM sequences [36, 69], and it signals similarly to other typical immunoreceptors, such as the antigen receptor of T lymphocytes (TCR) and the antigen receptor of B lymphocytes (BCR) [70]. The initial signaling steps for all immunoreceptors are alike and involve first cross-linking of the receptors on the membrane of the cell, followed by the activation of Src family tyrosine kinases (**Figure 4**). These kinases lead to activation of spleen tyrosine kinase (Syk), which in turn phosphorylates tyrosines within the ITAM sequence. Phosphorylated ITAM then becomes a binding site for Syk. After binding to the receptor, Syk phosphorylates multiple substrates leading to different cell responses [6, 31, 71] (**Figure 4**). Syk can phosphorylate and activate phospholipase Cγ (PLCγ), which in turn generates diacylglycerol (DAG) and inositol triphosphate (IP_3). DAG also activates protein kinase C (PKC), an important serine/threonine kinase that can lead to the activation of MAP kinases extracellular signal-regulated kinase (ERK) and p38 (**Figure 4**). IP_3 induces release of intracellular calcium from the endoplasmic reticulum. Calcium regulates several proteins such as calmodulin and calcineurin. Syk can also induce activation of phosphatidylinositol-3 kinase (PI3K), which produces phosphatidylinositol 3,4,5-trisphosphate (PIP_3). This phospholipid is relevant to the activation of small GTPases, such as Rho and Rac, which are involved in cytoskeleton remodeling for phagocytosis. Rac also leads to activation of the MAPK/ERK kinase (MEK)—ERK pathway, and to activation of c-Jun N-terminal kinases (JNK). These kinases are important for activation of nuclear factors, such as Elk-1, AP-1, and nuclear factor of activated T cells (NFAT) (**Figure 4**). These nuclear factors induce the expression of cytokines important for inflammation and immune regulation, such as IL-2, IL-6, IL-8, IL-10, tumor necrosis factor α (TNF-α), and IFN-γ [72–74] (**Figure 4**).

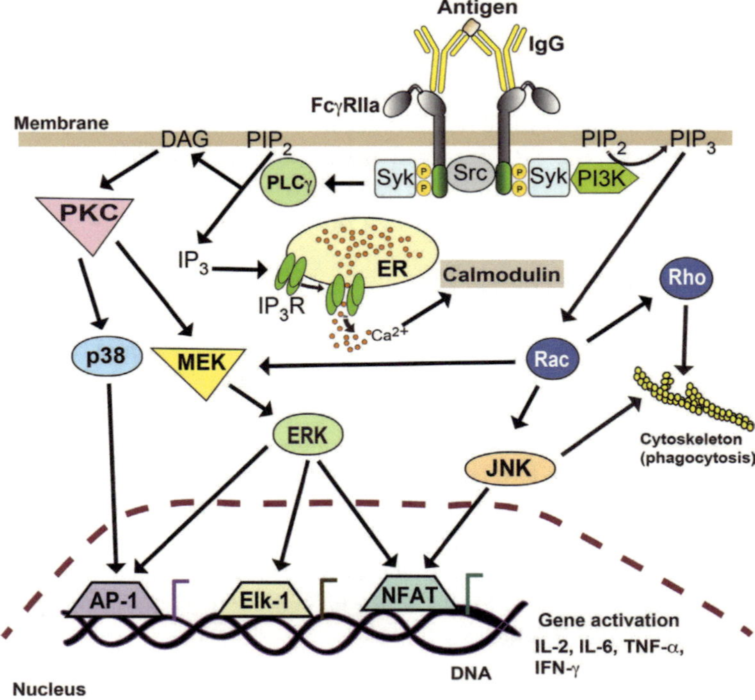

Figure 4.
Signaling transduction pathway of the neutrophil FcγRIIa. Engagement of activating FcγRIIa by IgG-antigen immune complexes induces receptor cross-linking and phosphorylation of tyrosine residues in the immunoreceptor tyrosine-based activation motif domains (green oval) by Src family kinases. Phosphorylated tyrosines then become docking sites for Syk, which in turn phosphorylates multiple substrates leading to different signaling pathways that ultimately activate various cell responses. See text for details. P represents a phosphate group; Syk, spleen tyrosine kinase; PI3K, phosphatidylinositol-3 kinase; PIP_2, phosphatidylinositol 4,5-bisphosphate; PIP_3, phosphatidylinositol 3,4,5-trisphosphate; JNK, c-Jun N-terminal kinase; NFAT, nuclear factor of activated T cells; PLCγ, phospholipase Cγ; DAG, diacylglycerol; IP_3, inositol triphosphate; IP_3R, receptor for IP_3; ER, endoplasmic reticulum; PKC, protein kinase C; MEK, MAPK/ERK kinase; ERK, extracellular signal-regulated kinase; p38, p38 MAP kinase; AP-1, activator protein 1; Elk-1, Ets LiKe gene1 (ETS) transcription factor; IL-2, interleukin-2; IL-6, interleukin-6; TNF-α, tumor necrosis factor α; and IFN-γ, interferon-γ.

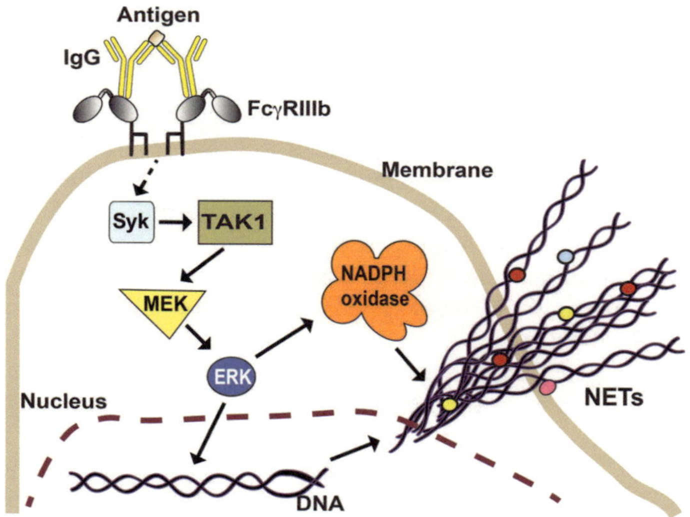

Figure 5.
Signaling transduction pathway of the neutrophil FcγRIIIb. Cross-linking of the human FcγRIIIb by IgG-antigen immune complexes induces activation of spleen tyrosine kinase (Syk) by a mechanism not yet described. Syk then activates transforming growth factor-β-activated kinase 1 (TAK1). TAK1 is in turn required for activation of ERK kinase (MEK) and extracellular signal regulated kinase (ERK). Activated ERK signals to the nucleus and contributes to activation of NADPH oxidase, which together lead to formation of neutrophil extracellular traps (NETs).

In contrast, the human FcγRIIIb is a GPI-linked receptor that lacks an intracellular portion. Thus, it is not clear how it can connect to intracellular signaling molecules. However, there is no doubt that FcγRIIIb is an activating receptor inducing several neutrophil responses such as increase in calcium concentration [75], activation of the respiratory burst [76], activation of integrins [77], and induction of NETosis [78, 79]. Despite, the initial signaling mechanism for FcγRIIIb remains unknown, the signaling pathway for this receptor engages Syk and then transforming growth factor-β-activated kinase 1 (TAK1), as well as the MEK/ERK cascade [80] (**Figure 5**). One possibility to connect FcγRIIIb with Syk is that the receptor could link with signaling molecules such as Src family tyrosine kinases on the plane of the cell membrane. Because GPI-linked proteins, like the FcγRIIIb, concentrate in lipid rafts on the cell membrane together with Src kinases [81, 82], we can imagine that after cross-linking FcγRIIIb, it associates somehow with these kinases and activates Syk. A possible connection is the binding of the receptor, within the lipid rafts, to a putative ITAM-containing molecule [83]. Many steps are still unknown and future research will help in completely elucidate this signaling pathway.

6. Each FcγR leads to unique cellular responses

The signaling pathways activated by immune complexes binding to Fcγ receptors stimulate different neutrophil responses including phagocytosis, respiratory burst, cytokine and chemokine production, and antibody-dependent cellular cytotoxicity (ADCC) [7, 8, 33]. However, our understanding of what particular function is activated in a cell responding to an individual type of FcγR is still very limited. This lack of knowledge is due, in part, to the fact that each cell expresses several types of FcγRs and all receptors can bind to more than one type of IgG. Thus, it is not clear whether each receptor leads to a particular response or the average signaling from various receptors activates a predetermined cell response. Traditionally, it has been thought that each cell is set to activate a particular cell function after FcγR cross-linking. More recently, however, another interpretation has been considered: each FcγR activates a particular signaling pathway leading to a unique cell response. In the traditional view, each cell is already programmed to perform a particular cell function after FcγR cross-linking, independently of the receptor used. This idea is not really supported by experimental evidence. As indicated above, different IgG subclasses bind particular Fcγ receptors with different affinity, leading to unique cell functions *in vivo* [42]. In the most recent view, each FcγR activates a distinctive signaling pathway leading to an individual cell function. This view is supported by recent reports, where individual FcγRs on human neutrophils initiate particular cell responses [77, 78, 84–86].

The idea that particular Fcγ receptors could activate unique cell functions was initially published more than 20 years ago. It was found that the neutrophil FcγRIIIb induced actin polymerization in a Ca^{2+}-dependent manner, while FcγRIIa did not [87]. This initial report was not followed by similar reports and the idea of one receptor one response was forgotten. However, with time, other reports have provided new evidence that supports this idea. Some years later, it was reported that FcγRIIa, but not FcγRIIIb caused shedding of L-selectin expression [88] (**Figure 6**). Consequently, it was proposed that binding of antibodies to FcγRIIIb could induce a proadhesive phenotype of neutrophils [88]. More recently, new evidence supporting this idea was found. When each receptor was selectively activated with specific monoclonal antibodies, FcγRIIIb but not FcγRIIa, was able to activate β1 integrins [77] (**Figure 7**). This activation resulted from an increase in binding affinity to fibronectin [77]. Thus, after neutrophils leave the circulation, engagement of FcγRIIIb could lead to activation β1 integrins, allowing the cells to adhere to extracellular matrix proteins and migrate into tissues [89] (**Figure 1**). In contrast, for antibody-mediated phagocytosis [17], FcγRIIa was the main Fcγ receptor mediating this response, while FcγRIIIb contribution to phagocytosis was minimal [86]. Therefore, at least in human neutrophils, each Fcγ receptor initiates particular cell functions. FcγRIIa induces phagocytosis (**Figure 6**), while FcγRIIIb promotes an adhesive phenotype via activation of β1 integrins (**Figure 7**).

In addition, it was also reported that FcγRIIIb signals to the neutrophil nucleus more efficiently than FcγRIIa. FcγRIIIb, but not FcγRIIa, induced a large increase

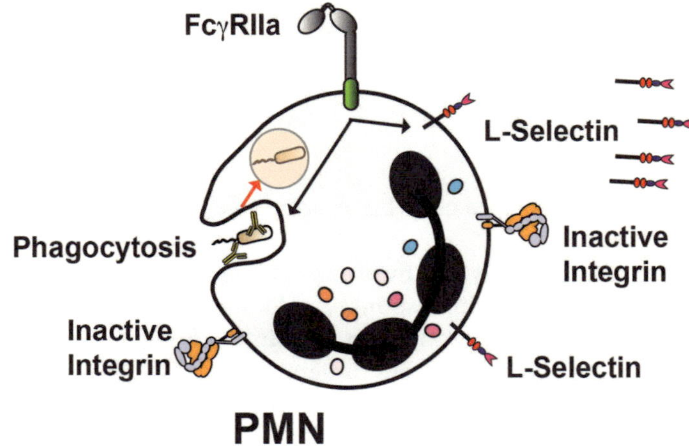

Figure 6.
Neutrophil functions activated by FcγRIIa. In human neutrophils, FcγRIIa signaling induces L-selectin shedding from the cell membrane, and also activates efficient phagocytosis. The oval represents IgG-opsonized bacteria.

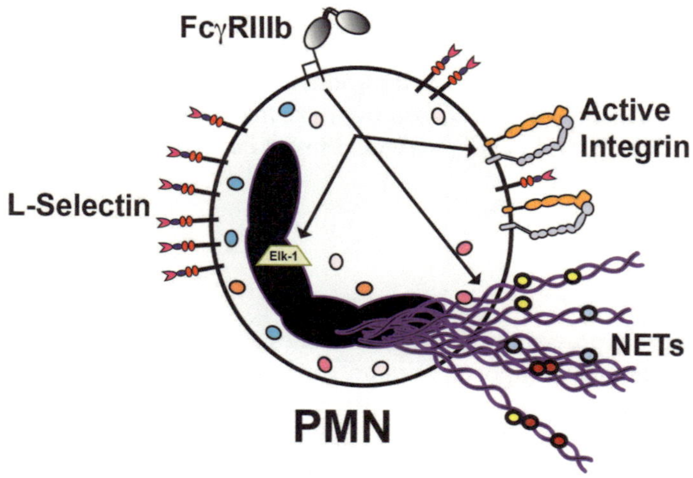

Figure 7.
Neutrophil functions activated by FcγRIIIb. Cross-linking of the human FcγRIIIb stimulates activation of β1 integrins promoting in this way a proadhesive neutrophil phenotype. FcγRIIIb also induces activation of the nuclear factor Elk-1 and formation of neutrophil extracellular traps (NETs).

in phosphorylated ERK in the nucleus, and also efficient phosphorylation of the nuclear factor Elk-1 [84] (**Figure 7**). Interestingly, FcγRIIa also induced phosphorylation of ERK in the cytosol [84, 90], but this active ERK seems to function mainly in enhancing phagocytosis and not in nuclear signaling [91] (**Figure 4**).

A recently discovered antimicrobial function of neutrophils is the formation of neutrophil extracellular traps (NETs) [92, 93]. NETs are induced by several pathogens, including virus, bacteria, fungi, and parasites [94]. Also, pro-inflammatory stimuli such as IL-8, TNF-α, and phorbol-12-myristate-13-acetate (PMA) are efficient inducers of NETs [95]. Because, antigen-antibody complexes are also capable of inducing NET formation [96]; it was clear that FcγRs were involved in NET formation. Recently, it was found that FcγRIIIb, but not FcγRIIa, is the receptor responsible for NET formation [78–80] (**Figure 8**).

Together, all these reports strongly reinforce the modern view that each FcγR induces a particular signaling pathway that activates a single cellular function. Elucidating the conditions that engage a single type of FcγR to activate a particular cellular response would be very helpful in the future for controlling some of cellular

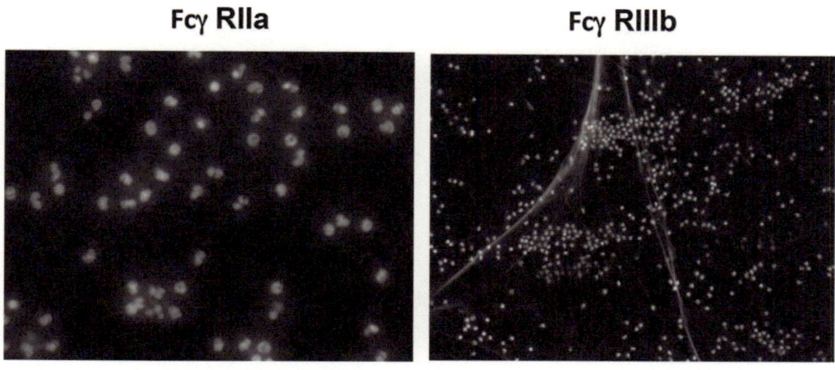

Figure 8.
Neutrophil FcγRIIIb, but not FcγRIIa, induces neutrophil extracellular traps (NETs) formation. Human neutrophils were stimulated by cross-linking FcγRIIa with the specific monoclonal antibody IV.3, or by cross-linking FcγRIIIb with the specific monoclonal antibody 3G8. After 4 hours, neutrophils were fixed and stained for DNA.

functions in clinical settings. For example, in intense infections, it may be important to activate phagocytosis. Because IgG2 binds better to FcγRIIa than to FcγRIIIb [33, 35], it is likely that IgG2 antibodies would activate phagocytosis by neutrophils much better than other IgG subclass antibodies. In consequence, promoting IgG2 antibodies against certain pathogens would result in better phagocytosis against them.

7. Conclusion

Fcγ receptors expressed in different immune cells are capable of activating different cellular responses important not only for controlling microbial infections but also for regulating immunity [71, 97]. Different subclasses of IgG antibodies bind the various Fcγ receptors with different affinities [33, 35] and can activate various cellular functions of great importance for host defense and for immune regulation. In the human neutrophil, it is clear that a specific Fcγ receptor activates particular cellular responses. FcγRIIa induces efficient phagocytosis [86], while FcγRIIIb signals to the nucleus for nuclear factor activation [84] and for NETs formation [78]. Therefore, in principle, a particular cell response could be induced or inhibited by engaging or blocking the corresponding FcγR. Information similar to the one described for neutrophil Fcγ receptors on other immune cells, such as monocytes or dendritic cells, is not available. Future research is needed in this area.

Acknowledgements

This work was supported by Grant 254434 from Consejo Nacional de Ciencia y Tecnología, México.

Author details

Carlos Rosales[1] and Eileen Uribe-Querol[2*]

1 Immunology Department, Instituto de Investigaciones Biomédicas, Universidad Nacional Autónoma de México, Mexico City, Mexico

2 Advanced Research Division, Facultad de Odontología, Universidad Nacional Autónoma de México, Mexico City, Mexico

*Address all correspondence to: euquerol@comunidad.unam.mx

References

[1] Mayadas TN, Cullere X, Lowell CA. The multifaceted functions of neutrophils. Annual Review of Pathology. 2014;**9**:181-218. DOI: 10.1146/annurev-pathol-020712-164023

[2] Tecchio C, Cassatella MA. Neutrophil-derived chemokines on the road to immunity. Seminars in Immunology. 2016;**28**:119-128. DOI: 10.1016/j.smim.2016.04.003

[3] Greenlee-Wacker MC. Clearance of apoptotic neutrophils and resolution of inflammation. Immunological Reviews. 2016;**273**:357-370. DOI: 10.1111/imr.12453

[4] Scapini P, Cassatella MA. Social networking of human neutrophils within the immune system. Blood. 2014;**124**:710-719. DOI: 10.1182/blood-2014-03-453217

[5] Nauseef WM, Borregaard N. Neutrophils at work. Nature Immunology. 2014;**15**:602-611. DOI: 10.1038/ni.2921

[6] Rosales C, Uribe-Querol E. Antibody—Fc receptor interactions in antimicrobial functions. Current Immunology Reviews. 2013;**9**:44-55. DOI: 10.2174/15733955113090 10006

[7] Rosales C, Uribe-Querol E. Fc receptors: Cell activators of antibody functions. Advances in Bioscience and Biotechnology. 2013;**4**:21-33. DOI: 10.4236/abb.2013.44A004

[8] Nimmerjahn F, Ravetch JV. FcγRs in health and disease. Current Topics in Microbiology and Immunology. 2011;**350**:105-125. DOI: 10.1007/82_2010_86

[9] Ravetch JV. Fc receptors. In: Paul WE, editor. Fundamental Immunology. 5th ed. Philadelphia: Lippincott Williams & Wilkins; 2003. pp. 631-684

[10] Borregaard N. Neutrophils, from marrow to microbes. Immunity. 2010;**33**:657-670. DOI: 10.1016/j.immuni.2010.11.011

[11] Deniset JF, Kubes P. Recent advances in understanding neutrophils. F1000Res. 2016;**5**:2912. DOI: 10.12688/f1000research.9691.1

[12] Kolaczkowska E, Kubes P. Neutrophil recruitment and function in health and inflammation. Nature Reviews. Immunology. 2013;**13**:159-175. DOI: 10.1038/nri3399

[13] Ley K, Laudanna C, Cybulsky M, Nourshargh S. Getting to the site of inflammation: The leukocyte adhesion cascade updated. Nature Reviews. Immunology. 2007;**7**:678-689. DOI: 10.1038/nri2156

[14] Arnaout MA. Biology and structure of leukocyte β2 integrins and their role in inflammation. F1000Res. 2016;**5** (F1000 Faculty Rev):2433. DOI: 10.12688/f1000research.9415.1

[15] Kourtzelis I, Mitroulis I, von Renesse J, Hajishengallis G, Chavakis T. From leukocyte recruitment to resolution of inflammation: The cardinal role of integrins. Journal of Leukocyte Biology. 2017;**102**:677-683. DOI: 10.1189/jlb.3MR0117-024R

[16] Gordon S. Phagocytosis: An immunobiologic process. Immunity. 2016;**44**:463-475. DOI: 10.1016/j.immuni.2016.02.026

[17] Rosales C, Uribe-Querol E. Phagocytosis: A fundamental process in immunity. BioMed Research International. 2017;**2017**:9042851. DOI: 10.1155/2017/9042851

[18] Jaumouillé V, Grinstein S. Molecular mechanisms of phagosome formation. Microbiology Spectrum. 2016;**4**: MCHD-0013-2015. DOI: 10.1128/microbiolspec.MCHD-0013-2015

[19] Levin R, Grinstein S, Canton J. The life cycle of phagosomes: Formation, maturation, and resolution. Immunological Reviews. 2016;**273**: 156-179. DOI: 10.1111/imr.12439

[20] Pham C. Neutrophil serine proteases: Specific regulators of inflammation. Nature Reviews. Immunology. 2006;**6**:541-550. DOI: 10.1038/nri1841

[21] Häger M, Cowland JB, Borregaard N. Neutrophil granules in health and disease. Journal of Internal Medicine. 2010;**268**:25-34. DOI: 10.1111/j. 1365-2796.2010. 02237.x

[22] Cowland JB, Borregaard N. Granulopoiesis and granules of human neutrophils. Immunological Reviews. 2016;**273**:11-28. DOI: 10.1111/imr.12440

[23] Sengeløv H, Follin P, Kjeldsen L, Lollike K, Dahlgren C, Borregaard N. Mobilization of granules and secretory vesicles during *in vivo* exudation of human neutrophils. Journal of Immunology. 1995;**154**:4157-4165

[24] Faurschou M, Borregaard N. Neutrophil granules and secretory vesicles in inflammation. Microbes and Infection. 2003;**5**:1317-1327. DOI: 10.1016/j.micinf.2003.09.008

[25] Branzk N, Lubojemska A, Hardison SE, Wang Q, Gutierrez MG, Brown GD, et al. Neutrophils sense microbe size and selectively release neutrophil extracellular traps in response to large pathogens. Nature Immunology. 2014;**15**:1017-1025. DOI: 10.1038/ni.2987

[26] Brinkmann V, Reichard U, Goosmann C, Fauler B, Uhlemann Y, Weiss DS, et al. Neutrophil extracellular traps kill bacteria. Science. 2004;**303**:1532-1535. DOI: 10.1126/science.1092385

[27] Fuchs TA, Abed U, Goosmann C, Hurwitz R, Schulze I, Wahn V, et al. Novel cell death program leads to neutrophil extracellular traps. The Journal of Cell Biology. 2007;**176**: 231-241. DOI: 10.1083/jcb.200606027

[28] Papayannopoulos V, Metzler KD, Hakkim A, Zychlinsky A. Neutrophil elastase and myeloperoxidase regulate the formation of neutrophil extracellular traps. The Journal of Cell Biology. 2010;**191**:677-691. DOI: 10.1083/jcb.201006052

[29] Björnsdottir H, Welin A, Michaëlsson E, Osla V, Berg S, Christenson K, et al. Neutrophil NET formation is regulated from the inside by myeloperoxidase-processed reactive oxygen species. Free Radical Biology & Medicine. 2015;**89**:1024-1035. DOI: 10.1016/j.freeradbiomed.2015. 10.398

[30] Ballow M. Historical perspectives in the diagnosis and treatment of primary immune deficiencies. Clinical Reviews in Allergy and Immunology. 2014;**46**:101-103. DOI: 10.1007/s12016-013-8384-9

[31] Rosales C. Fc receptor and integrin signaling in phagocytes. Signal Transduction. 2007;**7**:386-401. DOI: 10.1002/sita.200700141

[32] Heyman B. Regulation of antibody responses via antibodies, complement, and Fc receptors. Annual Review of Immunology. 2000;**18**:709-737. DOI: 10.1146/annurev.immunol.18.1.709

[33] Bruhns P, Jönsson F. Mouse and human FcR effector functions.

Immunological Reviews. 2015;**268**: 25-51. DOI: 10.1111/imr.12350

[34] Daëron M. Fc receptor biology. Annual Review of Immunology. 1997;**15**:203-234. DOI: 10.1146/annurev.immunol.15.1.203

[35] Bruhns P, Iannascoli B, England P, Mancardi D, Fernandez N, Jorieux S, et al. Specificity and affinity of human Fcγ receptors and their polymorphic variants for human IgG subclasses. Blood. 2009;**113**:3716-3725. DOI: 10.1182/blood-2008-09-179754

[36] Underhill DM, Goodridge HS. The many faces of ITAMs. Trends in Immunology. 2007;**28**:66-73. DOI: 10.1016/j.it.2006.12.004

[37] Stefanescu RN, Olferiev M, Liu Y, Pricop L. Inhibitory Fcγ receptors: From gene to disease. Journal of Clinical Immunology. 2004;**24**:315-326. DOI: 10.1023/B:JOCI.0000029105.47772.04

[38] Baerenwaldt A, Lux A, Danzer H, Spriewald BM, Ullrich E, Heidkamp G, et al. Fcγ receptor IIB (FcγRIIB) maintains humoral tolerance in the human immune system *in vivo*. Proceedings of the National Academy of Sciences of the United States of America. 2011;**108**:18772-18777. DOI: 10.1073/pnas.1111810108

[39] Daëron M, Lesourne R. Negative signaling in Fc receptor complexes. Advances in Immunology. 2006;**89**:39-86. DOI: 10.1016/S0065-2776(05)89002-9

[40] Nimmerjahn F, Ravetch J. Fcγ receptors as regulators of immune responses. Nature Reviews. Immunology. 2008;**8**:34-47. DOI: 10.1038/nri2206

[41] Lehmann B, Schwab I, Böhm S, Lux A, Biburger M, Nimmerjahn F. FcγRIIB: A modulator of cell activation and humoral tolerance. Expert Review of Clinical Immunology. 2012;**8**:243-254. DOI: 10.1586/eci.12.5

[42] Nimmerjahn F, Ravetch JV. Antibody-mediated modulation of immune responses. Immunological Reviews. 2010;**236**:265-275. DOI: 10.1111/j.1600-065X.2010.00910.x

[43] Willcocks LC, Smith KG, Clatworthy MR. Low-affinity Fcγ receptors, autoimmunity and infection. Expert Reviews in Molecular Medicine. 2009;**11**:e24. DOI: 10.1017/S1462399409001161

[44] Nimmerjahn F, Ravetch J. Fcγ receptors: Old friends and new family members. Immunity. 2006;**24**:19-28. DOI: 10.1016/j.immuni.2005.11.010

[45] Anthony RM, Wermeling F, Ravetch JV. Novel roles of the IgG Fc glycan. Annals of the New York Academy of Sciences. 2012;**1253**:170-180. DOI: 10.1111/j.1749-6632.2011.06305.x

[46] Raju T. Terminal sugars of Fc glycans influence antibody effector functions of IgGs. Current Opinion in Immunology. 2008;**20**:471-478. DOI: 10.1016/j.coi.2008.06.007

[47] Schroeder HWJ, Cavacini L. Structure and function of immunoglobulins. The Journal of Allergy and Clinical Immunology. 2010;**125**:S41-S52. DOI: 10.1016/j.jaci.2009.09.046

[48] Uchida J, Hamaguchi Y, Oliver J, Ravetch J, Poe J, Haas K, et al. The innate mononuclear phagocyte network depletes B lymphocytes through Fc receptor-dependent mechanisms during anti-CD20 antibody immunotherapy. The Journal of Experimental Medicine. 2004;**199**:1659-1669. DOI: 10.1084/jem.20040119

[49] Lambert S, Okada C, Levy R. TCR vaccines against a murine T cell lymphoma: A primary role for

antibodies of the IgG2c class in tumor protection. Journal of Immunology. 2004;**172**:929-936. DOI: 10.4049/jimmunol.172.2.929

[50] Nimmerjahn F, Bruhns P, Horiuchi K, Ravetch J. FcγRIV: A novel FcR with distinct IgG subclass specificity. Immunity. 2005;**23**:41-51. DOI: 10.1016/j.immuni.2005.05.010

[51] Nimmerjahn F, Ravetch J. Divergent immunoglobulin G subclass activity through selective Fc receptor binding. Science. 2005;**310**:1510-1512. DOI: 10.1126/science.1118948

[52] Wright A, Morrison SL. Effect of glycosylation on antibody function: Implications for genetic engineering. Trends in Biotechnology. 1997;**15**:26-32. DOI: 10.1016/S0167-7799(96) 10062-7

[53] Shields R, Namenuk A, Hong K, Meng Y, Rae J, Briggs J, et al. High resolution mapping of the binding site on human IgG1 for FcγRI, FcγRII, FcγRIII, and FcRn and design of IgG1 variants with improved binding to the FcγR. The Journal of Biological Chemistry. 2001;**276**:6591-6604. DOI: 10.1074/jbc.M009483200

[54] Arnold J, Wormald M, Sim R, Rudd P, Dwek R. The impact of glycosylation on the biological function and structure of human immunoglobulins. Annual Review of Immunology. 2007;**25**:21-50. DOI: 10.1146/annurev.immunol.25.022106.141702

[55] Jefferis R. Isotype and glycoform selection for antibody therapeutics. Archives of Biochemistry and Biophysics. 2012;**526**:159-166. DOI: 10.1016/j.abb.2012.03.021

[56] Mizuochi T, Taniguchi T, Shimitzu A, Kobata A. Structural and numerical variations of the carbohydrate moiety of immunoglobulin G. Journal of Immunology. 1982;**129**:2016-2020

[57] Shields R, Lai J, Keck R, O'Connell L, Hong K, Meng Y, et al. Lack of fucose on human IgG1 N-linked oligosaccharide improves binding to human FcγRIII and antibody-dependent cellular toxicity. The Journal of Biological Chemistry. 2002;**277**:26733-26740. DOI: 10.1074/jbc.M202069200

[58] Shinkawa T, Nakamura K, Yamane N, Shoji-Hosaka E, Kanda Y, Sakurada M, et al. The absence of fucose but not the presence of galactose or bisecting N-acetylglucosamine of human IgG1 complex-type oligosaccharides shows the critical role of enhancing antibody-dependent cellular cytotoxicity. The Journal of Biological Chemistry. 2003;**278**:3466-3473. DOI: 10.1074/jbc.M210665200

[59] Kubota T, Niwa R, Satoh M, Akinaga S, Shitara K, Hanai N. Engineered therapeutic antibodies with improved effector functions. Cancer Science. 2009;**100**:1566-1572. DOI: 10.1111/j.1349-7006.2009.01222.x

[60] Varki A. "Unusual" modifications and variations of vertebrate oligosaccharides: Are we missing the flowers from the trees? Glycobiology. 1996;**6**:707-710

[61] Kaneko Y, Nimmerjahn F, Ravetch J. Anti-inflammatory activity of immunoglobulin G resulting from Fc sialylation. Science. 2006;**313**:670-673. DOI: 10.1126/science.1129594

[62] Scallon B, Tam S, McCarthy S, Cai A, Raju T. Higher levels of sialylated Fc glycans in immunoglobulin G molecules can adversely impact functionality. Molecular Immunology. 2007;**44**:1524-1534. DOI: 10.1016/j.molimm.2006.09.005

[63] Anthony R, Wermeling F, Karlsson M, Ravetch J. Identification of a receptor required for the anti-inflammatory activity of IVIG. Proceedings of the National Academy of Sciences

of the United States of America. 2008;**105**:19571-19578. DOI: 10.1073/pnas.0810163105

[64] van Sorge NM, van der Pol WL, van de Winkel JG. FcγR polymorphisms: Implications for function, disease susceptibility and immunotherapy. Tissue Antigens. 2003;**61**:189-202. DOI: 10.1034/j.1399-0039.2003.00037.x

[65] Warmerdam PAM, van de Winkel JG, Gosselin EJ, Capel PAJ. Molecular basis for a polymorphism of human Fcγ receptor II (CD32). The Journal of Experimental Medicine. 1990;**172**:19-25. DOI: 10.1084/jem.172.1.19

[66] Huizinga TWJ, Kleijer M, Tetteroo PAT, Roos D, von dem Borne AEGK. Biallelic neutrophil Na-antigen system is associated with a polymorphism on the phospho-inositol-linked Fcγ receptor III (CD16). Blood. 1990;**75**:213-217

[67] Ory PA, Clark MR, Kwoh EE, Clarkson SB, Goldstein IM. Sequences of complementary DNAs that encode the NA1 and NA2 forms of Fc receptor III on human neutrophils. The Journal of Clinical Investigation. 1989;**84**: 1688-1691. DOI: 10.1172/JCI114350

[68] Bux J, Stein E-L, Bierling P, Fromont P, Clay M, Stroncek D, et al. Characterization of a new alloantigen (SH) on the human neutrophil Fcγ receptor IIIB. Blood. 1997;**89**: 1027-1034

[69] Fodor S, Jakus Z, Mócsai A. ITAM-based signaling beyond the adaptive immune response. Immunology Letters. 2006;**104**:29-37. DOI: 10.1016/j.imlet.2005.11.001

[70] Getahun A, Cambier JC. Of ITIMs, ITAMs, and ITAMis: Revisiting immunoglobulin Fc receptor signaling. Immunological Reviews. 2015;**268**: 66-73. DOI: 10.1111/imr.12336

[71] Bournazos S, Ravetch JV. Fcγ receptor pathways during active and passive immunization. Immunological Reviews. 2015;**268**:88-103. DOI: 10.1111/imr.12343

[72] Sánchez-Mejorada G, Rosales C. Signal transduction by immunoglobulin Fc receptors. Journal of Leukocyte Biology. 1998;**63**:521-533. DOI: 10.1002/jlb.63.5.521

[73] Mócsai A. Diverse novel functions of neutrophils in immunity, inflammation, and beyond. The Journal of Experimental Medicine. 2013;**210**:1283-1299. DOI: 10.1084/jem.20122220

[74] Uribe-Querol E, Rosales C. Neutrophils in cancer: Two sides of the same coin. Journal of Immunology Research. 2015;**2015**:983698. DOI: 10.1155/2015/983698

[75] Rosales C, Brown EJ. Signal transduction by neutrophil IgG Fc receptors: Dissociation of [Ca^{+2}] rise from IP_3. The Journal of Biological Chemistry. 1992;**267**:5265-5271

[76] Löfgren R, Serrander L, Forsberg M, Wilsson A, Wasteson A, Stendahl O. CR3, FcγRIIA and FcγRIIIB induce activation of the respiratory burst in human neutrophils: The role of intracellular Ca($^{2+}$), phospholipase D and tyrosine phosphorylation. Biochimica et Biophysica Acta. 1999;**1452**:46-59. DOI: 10.1016/S0167-4889(99)00112-3

[77] Ortiz-Stern A, Rosales C. FcγRIIIB stimulation promotes β1 integrin activation in human neutrophils. Journal of Leukocyte Biology. 2005;**77**:787-799. DOI: 10.1189/jlb.0504310

[78] Alemán OR, Mora N, Cortes-Vieyra R, Uribe-Querol E, Rosales C. Differential use of human neutrophil Fcγ receptors for inducing

neutrophil extracellular trap formation. Journal of Immunology Research. 2016;**2016**:142643. DOI: 10.1155/2016/2908034

[79] Behnen M, Leschczyk C, Möller S, Batel T, Klinger M, Solbach W, et al. Immobilized immune complexes induce neutrophil extracellular trap release by human neutrophil granulocytes via FcγRIIIB and Mac-1. Journal of Immunology. 2014;**193**:1954-1965. DOI: 10.4049/jimmunol.1400478

[80] Alemán OR, Mora N, Cortes-Vieyra R, Uribe-Querol E, Rosales C. Transforming growth factor-β-activated kinase 1 is required for human FcγRIIIb-induced neutrophil extracellular trap formation. Frontiers in Immunology. 2016;**7**:277. DOI: 10.3389/fimmu.2016.00277

[81] Reeves VL, Thomas CM, Smart EJ. Lipid rafts, caveolae and GPI-linked proteins. Adv. Exp. Med. Biol. 2012;**729**:3-13. DOI: 10.1007/978-1-4614-1222-9_1

[82] Paladino S, Lebreton S, Zurzolo C. Trafficking and membrane organization of GPI-anchored proteins in health and diseases. Current Topics in Membranes. 2015;**75**:269-303. DOI: 10.1016/bs.ctm.2015.03.006

[83] García-García E, Rosales C. Fc receptor signaling in leukocytes: Role in host defense and immune regulation. Current Immunology Reviews. 2009;**5**:227-242. DOI: 10.2174/157339509788921229

[84] García-García E, Nieto-Castañeda G, Ruiz-Saldaña M, Mora N, Rosales C. FcγRIIA and FcγRIIIB mediate nuclear factor activation through separate signaling pathways in human neuthophils. Journal of Immunology. 2009;**182**:4547-4556. DOI: 10.4049/jimmunol.0801468

[85] García-García E, Uribe-Querol E, Rosales C. A simple and efficient method to detect nuclear factor activation in human neutrophils by flow cytometry. Journal of Visualized Experiments. 2013;**74**:e50410. DOI: 10.3791/50410

[86] Rivas-Fuentes S, García-García E, Nieto-Castañeda G, Rosales C. Fcγ receptors exhibit different phagocytosis potential in human neutrophils. Cellular Immunology. 2010;**263**:114-121. DOI: 10.1016/j.cellimm.2010.03.006

[87] Salmon JE, Browle NL, Edberg JC, Kimberly RP. Fcγ receptor III induces actin polymerization in human neutrophils and primes phagocytosis mediated by Fcγ receptor II. Journal of Immunology. 1991;**146**:997-1004

[88] Kocher M, Siegel ME, Edberg JC, Kimberly RP. Cross-linking of Fcγ receptor IIa and Fcγ receptor IIIb induces different proadhesive phenotypes on human neutrophils. Journal of Immunology. 1997;**159**:3940-3948

[89] Ortiz-Stern A, Rosales C. Cross-talk between Fc receptors and integrins. Immunology Letters. 2003;**90**:137-143. DOI: 10.1016/j.imlet.2003. 08.004

[90] Coxon PY, Rane MJ, Powell DW, Klein JB, McLeish KR. Differential mitogen-activated protein kinase stimulation by Fcγ receptor IIa and Fcγ receptor IIIb determines the activation phenotype of human neutrophils. Journal of Immunology. 2000;**164**:6530-6537. DOI: 10.4049/jimmunol.164.12.6530

[91] Garcia-Garcia E, Rosales C. Adding complexity to phagocytic signaling: Phagocytosis-associated cell responses and phagocytic efficiency. In: Rosales C, editor. Molecular Mechanisms of Phagocytosis. Georgetown, Texas: Landes Bioscience/Springer Science; 2005. pp. 58-71

[92] Brinkmann V, Zychlinsky A. Beneficial suicide: Why neutrophils die to make NETs. Nature Reviews. Microbiology. 2007;**5**:577-582. DOI: 10.1038/nrmicro1710

[93] Yipp BG, Kubes P. NETosis: How vital is it? Blood. 2013;**122**:2784-2794. DOI: 10.1182/blood-2013-04-457671

[94] Branzk N, Papayannopoulos V. Molecular mechanisms regulating NETosis in infection and disease. Seminars in Immunopathology. 2013;**35**:513-530. DOI: 10.1007/s00281-013-0384-6

[95] Brinkmann V, Zychlinsky A. Neutrophil extracellular traps: Is immunity the second function of chromatin? The Journal of Cell Biology. 2012;**198**:773-783. DOI: 10.1083/jcb.201203170

[96] Short KR, von Köckritz-Blickwede M, Langereis JD, Chew KY, Job ER, Armitage CW, et al. Antibodies mediate formation of neutrophil extracellular traps in the middle ear and facilitate secondary pneumococcal otitis media. Infection and Immunity. 2014;**82**:364-370. DOI: 10.1128/IAI.01104-13

[97] Yu X, Lazarus AH. Targeting FcγRs to treat antibody-dependent autoimmunity. Autoimmunity Reviews. 2016;**15**:510-512. DOI: 10.1016/j.autrev.2016.02.006

Chapter 4

Remodeling of Phenotype $CD16^{+}CD11b^{+}$ Neutrophilic Granulocytes in Acute Viral and Acute Bacterial Infections

Irina V. Nesterova, Galina A. Chudilova, Svetlana V. Kovaleva, Lyudmila V. Lomtatidze and Tatyana V. Rusinova

Abstract

Neutrophilic granulocytes (NGs) are very important cells of innate immunity that can very quickly realize antibacterial and antiviral defense. Until the present time, the phenomenon of different levels of presentations of membrane receptors CD16 and CD11b NG in normal and pathological conditions wasn't studied. We had studied the population of $CD16^{+}CD11b^{+}$NG in two groups of patients with acute viral and acute bacterial infections in the models of acute bacterial tonsillitis (ABT) and acute viral tonsillitis-EBV infection (AEBVI), having the same clinical symptoms in early stages of the disease. Comparative analysis of the redistribution of equipment intensity of CD16 and CD11b has detected three subpopulations of $CD16^{+}CD11b^{+}$NG population—$CD16^{bright}CD11b^{bright}$, $CD16^{bright}CD11b^{dim}$, and $CD16^{dim}CD11b^{bright}$—in normal and pathological conditions. It was found that subpopulation $CD16^{bright}CD11b^{dim}$NG dominates in healthy individuals; subpopulation $CD16^{bright}CD11b^{bright}$NG dominates in patients with acute viral infection; subpopulation $CD16^{dim}CD11b^{bright}$NG dominates in patients with acute bacterial infections. We had demonstrated that the study of $CD16^{+}CD11b^{+}$NG subpopulations allows in early stage of diseases to diagnose acute viral and acute bacterial infections. Our studies have demonstrated the positive effects of eukaryotic DNA sodium salt on the negatively altered phenotype subpopulation $CD16^{+}CD11b^{+}$NG, in particular, through the remodeling of the expression of CD11b on NG membrane.

Keywords: neutrophilic granulocytes, subset, phenotype, receptors, acute viral and bacterial infections, eukaryotic DNA sodium salt

1. Introduction

Neutrophil granulocytes (NGs) are the most mobile and numerous populations of innate immunity cell, which reacts lightly to any aggression, which also carries out powerful anti-infectious protection.

The surprising universality and multifunctionality of this cell, once again, underline the existence of heterogeneity within the NG population, that is, the presence of subpopulations with different immunological roles. The use of monoclonal antibodies made it possible to confirm the existence of NG subpopulations using phenotypic characteristics. In 1998, the first nomenclature of human neutrophils antigens (HNAs) was created on the basis of membrane-expressed glycoprotein groups: HNA-1 (FcγRIIIb, CD16), HNA-2 (CD177), HNA-3 (CTL2), HNA-4 (CD11b/CD18, Mac-1, CR3), and HNA-5 (CD11a/CD18) [1]. The concept of heterogeneity of NG was discussed by scientists for more than 20 years and was confirmed with the accumulation of evidence on the presence of subsets of NG with various functions both in healthy subjects and in various diseases. Various methods have been used to detect the subpopulations of NG, such as cell maturity, functional activity, and localization, including receptors or markers of the cell surface.

2. Neutrophil granulocyte receptors

Cell populations and subpopulations of NG show a high degree of plasticity and functional heterogeneity depending on the characteristics of the course of physiological or pathological scenarios of the immune response, which, first of all, is due to potent receptor equipment. The membrane complex of NG expresses adhesion molecules, receptors for different ligands: cytokines, immunoglobulins, other cell membrane molecules, etc. NGs are capable to express MHC-1, selectins (CD62L), selectin receptors (CD162 (PSGL-1)), integrins (CD18 (β2-integrin), CD11a (LFA-1), CD11b (CR3), CD11c (CR4), CD11d), integrin receptors (ICAM receptors for β2-integrins - ICAM-1 (CD50), ICAM-3 (CD54). NG expresses receptors for chemoattractants (PFPR and FPLR for fMLP), receptors for chemokines (CXCR1, CXC2, CCR1), FcR receptors (CD16 (FcγRIII), CD32 (FcγRII), CD64 (FcγRI), CD89 (FcαRI), FcεR), receptors for complement components (CR1 (CD35), CR3 (CD11b), CR4 (CD11c), C5aR, C3aR, C5L2), receptor for LPS and endotoxins (CD14), cell adhesion receptor (CD15). NG receptors are involved in binding bacteria, in angiogenesis and apoptosis (CD17), in cell proliferation and differentiation (CD24), in PAMP recognition (TLR 1, 2, 4-10; NOD - receptors). In addition, on NG membrane there is a costimulatory receptor for B- lymphocytes (CD28), apoptosis activation/induction receptor (CD95), IL-2 receptor (CD25), which is NG activation marker; there are also molecules that determine the ability of NG to be APC (CD40, CD80, CD86, MHC II). NGs have multiple receptors for cytokines (IL-8, TNFα, IL-1, IL-2, IL-15, IL-17, IFNα, IFNγ, G-CSF, GM-CSF, etc.), hormones, neuropeptides, histamine, and kinases. The recently revealed expression of TCR-like (TCRL, TCRαβ) receptors on NG membrane, present throughout the life of a person and decreasing in old age, opens up new, previously unknown immune mechanisms for the functioning of NG [2] (**Figure 1**).

NGs are equipped with receptors that recognize endogenous molecules of "danger" alarms or danger-associated molecular patterns (DAMPs)—extracellular ATP, fragments of the extracellular matrix, heat shock proteins, nucleic acids (DNA and RNA fragments of its own cells), nuclear protein HMGB-1, and others—through which activation of the cell takes place and its inclusion in the inflammation reaction [3]. It has been established that the initiation of apoptosis of NG in clinically healthy individuals is under the influence of TNFα, sTRAIL, and IL-4 ligand [4]. Recently, new ways of activating the NG signal via ITAM/Syk-CARD9 have been described in the interaction of β-glycans with dectin-1, which triggers the synthesis of the cytokine IL-23 inducing the formation of Th17 cells [5]. NG receptor pool is located on intracellular membrane of secretory vesicles, gelatinase and specific granules, these receptors are translocated to surface membrane of NG only under the action of inducing stimuli [6]. Thus, the membrane expression of NG not only reflects the

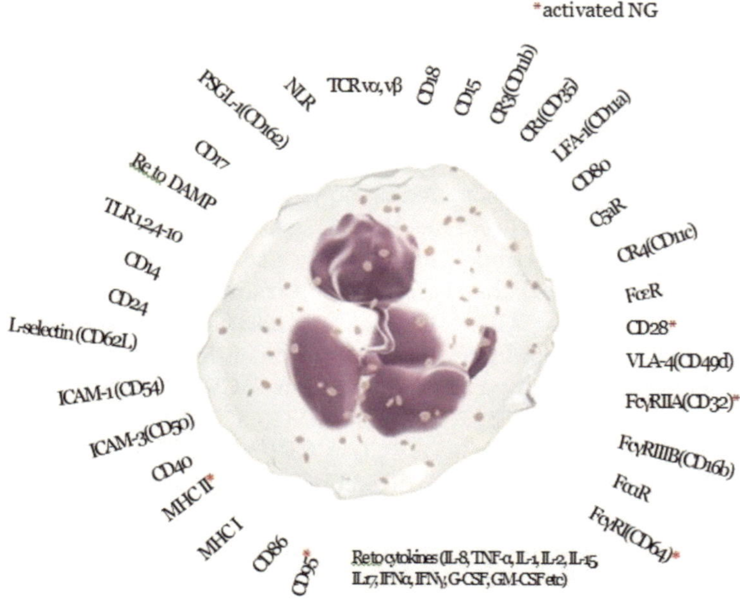

Figure 1.
Surface membrane receptors of neutrophilic granulocytes.

processes occurring during the life cycle of the cell but also allows us to evaluate the functional priming by reorganizing the surface cytoplasmic membrane of NG.

3. Phenotypic profile and functional features of neutrophil granulocytes

The study of the subpopulations of NG presents a new approach to the determination of functional activity of NG, allowing to assess the adequacy of the inclusion of NG in the implementation of the immune response, as well as to diagnose and predict the outcome of the disease. It is known that various phenotypic profiles and the level of equipment with surface receptors are associated with morphological features and determine the functional potential of NG-cytokine production, transendothelial migration, intracellular and extracellular killing, and formation of NET [7–9]. The existence of a sufficiently large number of NG subpopulations with different possibilities is demonstrated. NGs that receive complex cytokine influences not only acquire new features but also undergo different stages of activation and differentiation while expressing MHCII antigens, CD80, CD86, ICAM-1, and LFA-1 [7, 10, 11]. It has been shown that inducing cytokine stimuli differentiates NG in a unique hybrid subpopulation with dual phenotypic and functional properties characteristic of both NG and dendritic cells (DC) involved in innate and adaptive immune responses [12]. We have identified in our earlier works the following subpopulations of NG: regulatory; suppressor; pro-inflammatory, initiating inflammatory reaction; inflammatory with a positive microbicidal potential (antibacterial, antiviral, antifungal); inflammatory with negative cytotoxic potential, “aggressive”; anti-inflammatory, regulating inflammation regression; antineoplastic, TAN1; and pro-tumor, TAN2 and hybrid [13]. Phagocytic and microbicidal function and virucidal activity of NG are directly dependent on phenotypic features: the number and density of such expressed receptors as CD11b/CD18, CD10, CD15, CD16, CD32, CD64, CD35, etc. [6]. Expression on NG membrane of CD32 and CD16 is important in the realization of phagocytic function and antibody-dependent cellular cytotoxicity (ADCC), which is associated with CD11b-/CD18-dependent enhancement of adhesion, degranulation, and killing [14]. CD64, CD32, and CD16 are triggering molecules that induce immune phagocytosis and killing processes [15].

The variants of remodeling of NG phenotype simultaneously expressing functionally significant receptors CD64, CD32, CD11b, and CD16 in patients with infectious and inflammatory diseases, including newborns of different gestational ages [15], patients with neoplastic processes [10, 16], women of reproductive age with genital and extragenital infectious-inflammatory diseases [17] have great diagnostic and prognostic significance. When we study the variability of the simultaneous presentation of NG receptors CD64, CD32, CD16, and CD11b on the membrane, it was established that in healthy adults and children of different ages in the peripheral blood, there is one major subpopulation of $CD64^{-}CD32^{+}CD16^{+}CD11b^{+}$ and five minor subpopulations of NG, $CD64^{-}CD32^{+}CD16^{+}CD11b^{-}$, $CD64^{-}CD32^{-}CD16^{+}CD11b^{+}$, $CD64^{+}CD32^{+}CD16^{+}CD11b^{+}$, $CD64^{+}CD32^{+}CD16^{+}CD11b^{-}$, and $CD64^{+}CD32^{-}CD16^{+}CD11b^{+}$, with different equipment and density of studied receptors. We detected a significant increase in NG subpopulation with $CD64^{+}CD32^{+}CD16^{+}CD11b^{+}$ phenotype with a high expression density of CD11b and CD16 in newborns with infectious and inflammatory diseases of bacterial etiology (congenital pneumonia, neonatal sepsis) (**Figure 2**).

The observed increase in this subpopulation of NG in the peripheral blood is directly related to the severity of the infectious-inflammatory process: the more clinically severe the disease, the greater the number of NG with this phenotype $CD64^{+}CD32^{+}CD16^{+}CD11b^{+}$ is in circulation [18]. In fertile age women with genital and extragenital infectious and inflammatory diseases planning pregnancy, the phenotypic variability of NG—the appearance of a subpopulation of $CD16^{+}CD32^{+}$CD11b—was also revealed, which indicates a persistent violation of their receptor function and the need for its adequate correction consisting in restoring the phenotypic composition of NG. Thus, the provision of pre-gravity training with the inclusion of immunotherapy has a positive clinical and immunological effect, which consists in normalizing the receptor function of NG, which

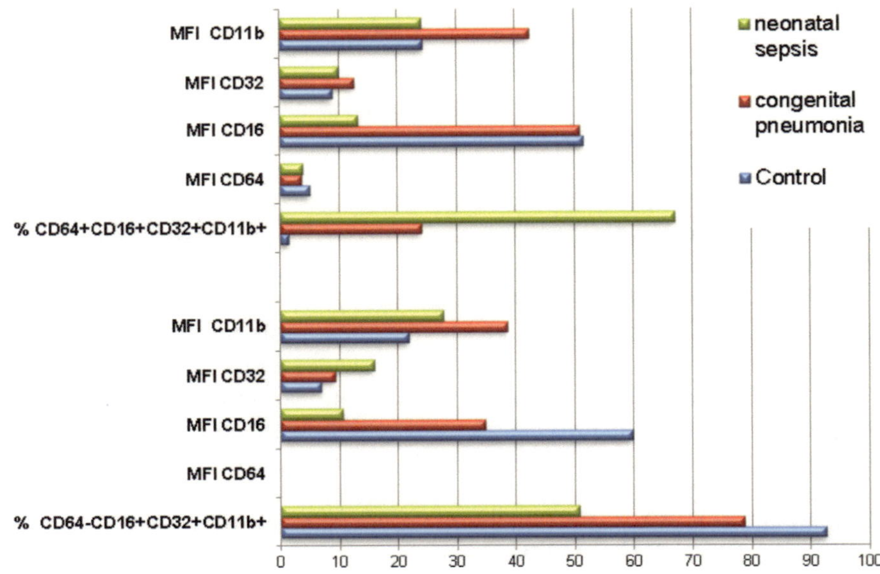

Figure 2.
Phenotypic profiles of $CD64^{+}CD32^{+}CD16^{+}CD11b^{+}$ NG in children with congenital pneumonia and neonatal sepsis.

correlates with an increase in the percentage of women who become pregnant [17]. The obtained data allow us to develop criteria for monitoring the course of associated viral infections and bacterial pro-inflammatory diseases, to diagnose and/or predict the aggravation of their severity, and to optimize immunotherapy methods aimed at correcting NG dysfunction. Multiple increases in the subpopulation of $CD64^-CD32^-CD16^+CD11b^+$ NG have been shown in children with repeated acute respiratory viral infections associated with herpesviral mono- or mixed infection. There was a significant replicative activity of herpesviruses such as HSV I/HSV II, CMV, EBV, and HHV VI [18, 19]. In addition, authors of this article put together all information into the table for the period from 2010 to 2016, about NG subpopulation phenotype according to their studies (**Table 1**).

Specific NG subpopulation composition and also adequate level of corresponding surface membrane marker expression density is important for the proper NG function. Thus, Pillay et al. found several subpopulations of NG with different phenotypes, which differed in the number and density of equipment with receptors: mature NG with the phenotype $CD16^{high}CD62L^{high}$, immature NG with the phenotype $CD16^{low}CD62L^{high}$, suppressive NG with the phenotype $CD16^{high}CD62L^{low}$, and NG precursors with the phenotype $CD16^{low}CD62L^{low}$ [11]. Circulating NG subpopulation with the phenotype $CD16^{low}CD62L^{high}$ was observed in children with respiratory syncytial viral infection, as well as in viral and bacterial coinfection

Group	Subpopulation	Functions/diagnostic significance
Healthy adults and children	$CD64^-CD32^+CD16^+CD11b^+$ $CD16^{bright}CD11b^{dim}$ $CD62L^{bright}CD63^{dim}$ $CD62L^{dim}CD63^{dim}$ (1:1)	-Anti-inflammatory and antitumor effect
		-Major subpopulations in healthy individuals -Full implementation of ADCC, microbicidal activity
Purulent-septic diseases in children and adults	$CD64^+CD32^+CD16^+CD11b^+$ $CD62L^{dim}CD63^{mid}$ $CD62L^{dim}CD63^{dim}$	-Marker of severity of bacterial infection process
		- Minor subpopulation in healthy individuals - Activated NG in vivo by bacterial antigens (significant increase in circulation)
Acute bacterial infection in adults	$CD16^{dim}CD11b^{bright}$	-Marker of acute process of the bacterial infection
		- Major subpopulation (significant increase in circulation)
Respiratory and herpes infections in children	$CD64^-CD16^+CD32^-CD11b^+$	-Prognostic sign of adverse course of viral infection
		- Minor subpopulation in healthy individuals -Significant increase at viral respiratory and herpetic infection - Depression of NG phagocytic and microbicidal activity
Acute EBV infection in adults	$CD16^{bright}CD11b^{bright}$	- Marker of severity of viral infection process - Prognostic sign of concomitant bacterial infection
		- Major subpopulation (significant increase in circulation) - High level of ADCC reaction and ROS-dependent inhibition of T-cell proliferation

Table 1.
Neutrophilic granulocyte subpopulation phenotypes and their function and diagnostic significance (Nesterova I.V. et al., 2010–2016).

[20, 21]. It is shown that the subpopulation of immature NG did not possess the ability to protect against microorganisms. Activated mature NG with immunosuppressive properties was found in patients with HIV infection [22]. Suppressive NG can cause paralysis of the immune system, as a result of which anti-infective protection is disrupted, which facilitates the occurrence of bacterial complications and the emergence of viral and bacterial coinfection [20, 23]. The appearance of $CD16^{high}CD62L^{low}$ NG significantly increases with bacterial infection or viral and bacterial coinfection, and at the same time, in the lower respiratory tract, in lungs this subpopulation is practically not detected in patients with viral infection [11, 20]. Neutrophilic subpopulation characterized by the phenotype $CD16^{low}CD62L^{low}$ was observed in children with severe viral respiratory infection without bacterial coinfection and in patients with bacterial sepsis [20, 21]. Using flow cytometry in combination with a visual evaluation of cells, it was shown that a large number of myelocytes and metamyelocytes are included in this subpopulation, so NG with the phenotype $CD16^{low}CD62L^{low}$ was called a subpopulation of NG precursors. A sequential increase in the number of NG precursors was statistically significant ($p < 0.001$) and did not depend on the presence of bacterial coinfection [20]. It was suggested that the NG precursors originate from a heterogeneous family of granulocyte myeloid-derived suppressor cells (G-MDSCs), which include granulocyte cells with the property of immune inhibition [20, 24]. Significant differences in the number of markers of activation and degranulation of CD11b, CD54, CD63, and CD66b in the above four subpopulations (mature NG, immature NG, suppressor NG, and NG "precursors") in viral infections and in bacterial coinfections in newborns with severe viral infection, practically, are not revealed. It was noted that the activation and degranulation of suppressor NG revealed a high level of expression of CD11b and CD63, whereas in NG "precursors," the highest level of expression of CD63 and CD66b and a low level of expression of CD11b and CD54 were observed [20]. Interestingly that NG number in the bloodstream equipped with CD62L on the surface membrane is larger than CD62L NG obtained from bronchoalveolar lavage, which is presumably associated with the loss of this receptor during migration. Pillay et al. [11, 24] discovered the existence of a new subpopulation $CD11c^{bright}CD62L^{dim}CD16^{bright}CD11b^{bright}$ NG—mature hypersegmented human NG with immunosuppressive activity. This subpopulation was able to suppress the proliferation of T cells through the release of active forms of the oxygenate and showed high expression of CD11b. Earlier studies by Woodfin A. and co-authors demonstrated that suppressive NGs—mature cells with hypersegmented nucleus, expressing high levels of ICAM-1—have the ability to reverse transendothelial migration (TEM) [25]. Later, Cortjens and his colleagues in 2017 [20] showed that in severe respiratory viral infection in infants, the expression of the activation marker CD11b was significantly increased in the suppressor subpopulation of NG. These suppressor subpopulations of NG, which appeared in viral and bacterial coinfections in newborns, also had the highest expression of CD63 molecules on surface membranes, which indicated active degranulation of NG.

4. Neutrophil granulocytes in infectious diseases

Defective functioning NGs (deficiency of NG amount; violation of phagocytic function; deficiency of myeloperoxidase, defensins, lactoferrin, glucose-6-phosphate dehydrogenase, NADPH oxidase, etc.; defects in the formation of NET) do not provide adequate antimicrobial protection, which leads to the development of atypically occurring infectious and inflammatory diseases, sepsis, acute hematogenous osteomyelitis, recurrent purulent infections, chronic bacterial infections, etc. Adequate response of NG in contact with various aggressive pathogens (viruses, bacteria, fungi) can develop in different ways. At the same time, the lack of functional activity of NG is a risk factor for the development of many pathological conditions. Changes in both quantitative and functional characteristics of different subsets of NG are recorded in pathological conditions, that is, NG phenotype is transformed due to a multivariate change in the expression of various receptors. In this case, the defectiveness of microbicidal and regulatory functions of NG leads to a violation of antigen elimination and, as a result, to the aggravation of the course of acute or chronic bacterial, viral, and fungal infections [13]. At present, various dysfunctions of NG are described, which can proceed according to different scenarios in patients with infectious diseases with atypical current: (1) hypofunction and NG deficiency in recurrent and persistent-relapsing purulent processes and chronic infectious diseases, viral and bacterial etiology, not amenable to standard treatment; (2) blockade of functional activity of NG, manifested by the development of an inadequate response up to the state of non-response in chronic sluggish infectious and inflammatory processes with a protracted course of exacerbations in socially significant infections and sepsis; and (3) hyperfunctioning of NG (e.g., extracellular production of oxygen radicals in a high concentration), which can lead to suppression of the T cells and other members of the immune system and damage different organs and tissues in chronic immune-dependent diseases or septic shock [26–28]. Atypically occurring infectious and inflammatory diseases against the background of immune system disorders, and, in particular, against the background of NG dysfunction, lead to increased morbidity, partial and sometimes complete loss of ability to work, and high lethality in sepsis, both in adult subjects and in children especially in the neonatal period [29, 30].

Neonatal NG characterized qualitative and quantitative deficit compared to adult NG. Neonatal sepsis is a global problem because it has the most severe consequences and is characterized by high mortality. This occurs against the background of impairments in the functioning of the immune system and defective NG, which contributes to the rapid dissimilation of the infection and, as a result, to the death of the newborn [31]. Thus, three important violations of NG that contribute to the emergence of severe neonatal sepsis and septic shock are described: neutropenia, decreased plasticity, and delayed apoptosis [32]. In the case of sepsis or the syndrome of a systemic inflammatory reaction, a large number of immature forms of NG appear in circulation. NGs are characterized by a decrease in phagocytic functional activity, a decreased production of ROS, a defective expression level of CD14 receptors, and a violation of the migratory ability. Immature NGs are characterized by a high basal level of intracellular TNF-α/IL-10 ratio, which confirms their pro-inflammatory phenotype. They have a longer life cycle, are resistant to spontaneous apoptosis, and can mature ex vivo [33]. Patients with sepsis (a more severe inflammatory reaction) have a more pronounced decrease in some receptors, in particular TREM-1, which has a key role in amplifying the production of inflammatory cytokines than patients suffering from a noninfectious systemic inflammatory reaction syndrome [34].

NGs affect the adaptive immune response in viral infection [13, 22] through antigen presentation, translocation of pathogenic viruses to the lymph nodes, suppressor modulation of the T-cell response, and expression of Toll-like receptors recognizing the herpesvirus DNA (TLR-9) [35–37]. NGs are important elements of antiviral immunity, realizing their capabilities through the process of phagocytosis, the formation of active forms of oxygen (ROS), the formation of NET, and the ability to synthesize and secrete cytokines, defensins, and interferons [18, 38–40]. Recent studies have shown that on the one hand, NG can perform antiviral protection and on the other hand, many viruses, in particular herpesviruses, can negatively affect the function of the NG, transform their phenotype, and influence the formation of populations/subpopulations with different functional properties [22]. Herpes viruses block NG antiviral activity, increase NG apoptosis, which leads to neutropenia. Damage to the NG by herpesviruses disrupts their functioning and leads in combination with other factors to disruption of adaptation reactions [13, 22, 36, 41, 42]. In recent years, it has been shown that in chronic herpesviral infection, there are numerous subpopulations of the NG, characterized by different phenotypes with different receptor equipment, possessing different functional properties: the ability to restructure chromatin, express cytokine genes and secrete cytokines, realize the activity of the granular apparatus, produce active oxygen species, and form NET and cytotoxicity.

4.1 $CD16^+CD11b^+$ phenotype of neutrophilic granulocytes in acute viral and acute bacterial infections

The first reports of the heterogeneity of CD16 expression (FcγIII) on NG membrane (induces oxidative burst and phagocytosis) appeared more than 25 years ago [25, 43, 44], but only recently the mechanisms and functional consequences of this heterogeneity have been studied. In particular we have identified different $CD16^+CD11b^+$ NG phenotypes with individual characteristics in patients with acute viral (acute viral Epstein-Barr (EBV) infection) and acute bacterial infectious-inflammatory diseases (acute bacterial tonsillitis) [45]. Summarizing the obtained data, it should be noted that in healthy subjects, $CD16^{bright}CD11b^{dim}$NG subpopulation was major. The NG of this subpopulation in trace amounts was detected with acute viral infection and was completely absent in acute bacterial infection. In acute viral infection, the number of NGs of a highly equipped subpopulation—$CD16^{bright}CD11b^{bright}$NG—significantly increased, whereas in acute bacterial infection, there was a significantly lower increase in the number of NGs of this subpopulation. At the same time, in healthy individuals the subpopulation of $CD16^{bright}CD11b^{bright}$NG was minor. In the case of acute bacterial infection, the $CD16^{dim}CD11b^{bright}$ NG subpopulation, which was absent in conditionally healthy individuals, became dominant, and in the case of acute viral infection, it appeared in an insignificant amount. Subpopulation $CD16^{dim}CD11b^{dim}$ was detected only in healthy individuals (**Figure 3**).

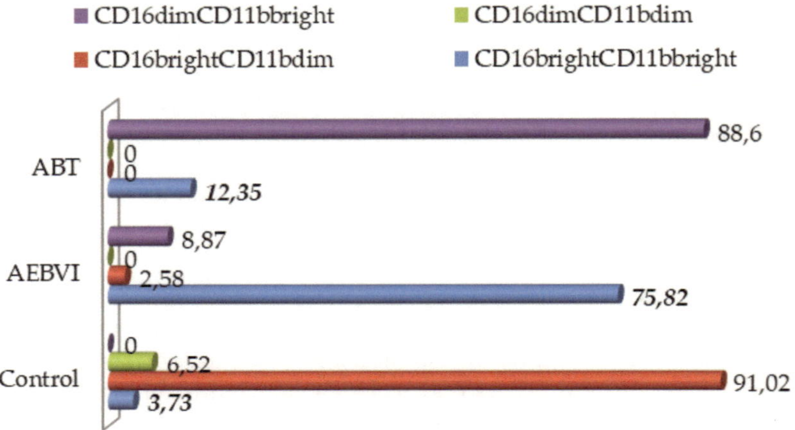

Figure 3.
Phenotypic profiles of $CD16^+CD11b^+$NG in acute viral (AEBVI) and acute bacterial (ABT) infections.

Apparently, this is a reserve nonactivated pool of circulating NG, since it is known that in the resting state, the NG is insignificantly equipped with membranes CD16 and CD11b. It should be noted that there are certain difficulties and differences in interpreting the data concerning the reasons for the low equipment of the NG CD16 receptor. Thus, early works of Elghetany M. T. (2002) [6] states that, in inflammation, the expression level of CD16 decreases and explain this phenomenon by shading this receptor; then Elghetany and Lacombe note that surface antigen expression of granulocytes depends on age, sex, race, and the presence of stress [46]. Pillay et al. [24] noted the appearance of a "paradoxical" NG population of low-membrane CD16-CD16^{dim} NG in the experiment with the introduction of LPS in vivo. The authors linked this phenomenon to the release of immature forms of granulocytes in the blood, reinforcing this conclusion with morphological studies: CD16^{dim}NG demonstrates the morphology of "young" band nuclear NG [47]. Thus, it is possible that the appearance of the prevalent major population of CD16^{dim}CD11b^{bright} in the acute bacterial infection of the pharyngeal lymphoid ring in patients in a state of moderate severity or with a severe condition is associated with the release of immature forms of the NG into circulation, which is a stereotype response of the NG in severe bacterial infection. The predominant subpopulation of CD16^{bright}CD11b^{bright}NG in patients with acute viral infection has a high cytotoxic antiviral potential due to the high level of CD16 and CD11b expression. According to Kushner and Cheung [48], the detectable enhanced expression of CD16 on NG in a viral infection may be due to the greater functional significance of cytotoxic NGs expressing FcγRIII (CD16) for the implementation of ADCC associated with CD11b-dependent increase in adhesion and degranulation [14].

The clinical picture of many infectious diseases of viral or bacterial etiology in the early stages of the disease can proceed according to a similar scenario. In this case, when verifying the diagnosis of an acute infectious process of viral or bacterial etiology, there are often certain difficulties that prevent timely proper selection of etiotropic therapy. Conducting an express analysis that allows us to specify dominant NG subpopulation—CD16^{bright}CD11b^{bright} or CD16^{dim}CD11b^{bright} can contribute to the differential diagnosis of acute viral and acute bacterial processes of the lymphogenous ring, which will allow timely optimization of etiotropic therapy. On the other hand, it is possible that the evaluation of these subpopulations of NG can be used for early differential diagnosis of various acute viral and acute bacterial processes of other localizations; however, this requires further study.

Thus, CD16^{bright}CD11b^{dim} NG subpopulations prevail in healthy subjects from 80 and up to 99.9%. In acute viral infection of the lymphogenous ring—infectious mononucleosis associated with EBV—the predominance of the subpopulation CD16^{bright}CD11b^{bright}NG is detected in an amount of 40% or more. In acute bacterial infection of the lymphatic pharynx, a subpopulation CD16^{dim}CD11b^{bright} NG predominates—from 40% and higher. The observed phenomenon of different dynamics of presentation of CD16 and CD11b membrane receptors in the CD16^{+}CD11b^{+} NG population in healthy individuals and acute inflammation in the region of the lymphopharynx ring reflects the differentiated response of NG to acute viral and acute bacterial infections.

4.2 Evaluation of the effects of the sodium salt of eukaryotic DNA and ODN2395 on CD16^{+}CD11b^{+}NG phenotype in patients with acute viral and bacterial infection

The use of drugs to improve the accuracy of exposure to target cells and selectively trigger the type of effector reaction is currently considered topical;

in particular, the use of exogenous oligomers of RNA and DNA, in the process of metabolism of which nucleotides and deoxynucleotides are formed, is promising [49]. Nucleic acid preparations of immunomodulating action of various natures are widely used in practical medicine. Pharmacopoeial preparations are known: sodium nucleate (RNA derived from yeast) [50], sodium deoxyribonucleate (sodium salt of native DNA isolated from sturgeon fish milt) [51], and placentex-integro (DNA from trout milt) [52]. Now, the team of authors [49] showed that the substance of sodium deoxyribonucleate mainly contains short and medium DNA chains ending in the CpG motif. Recognition of CpG motifs by the immune system occurs through their interaction with the Toll-like receptor 9 (TLR9), which acts on the cells as "alarm," activating innate and acquired immunity and many times enhancing the body's response even to low-immunogenic antigens [53] with effects of increased proliferation, maturation, and secretion of a number of biologically active molecules—cytokines, costimulatory molecules, molecules of the main histocompatibility complex, etc. [51, 54]. Inflammation is directly related to neutrophilic granulocytes (NGs), which express almost all known TLRs [55], which explains their crucial role in the regulation of phagocytic cells. It should be noted that activation of TLR-4 induces e production of pro-inflammatory cytokines and chemokines (IL1β, IL8, TNFα), TLR-2 activation induces production of chemokine MCP-1, and synchronous activation of TLR-4 and TLR-9 is accompanied by a pronounced respiratory burst a change in the expression of NG adhesion molecules [56, 57]. In the current literature, there are data on the cooperation of TLR9 with the functionally significant receptor of phagocytes—CD11b in the process of recognition of pathogens, even at a low level of exposure to such pathogens [58]. CD11b is also known to both positively and negatively regulate TLR9-mediated mechanisms: control TLR9-triggered NK cell cytotoxicity and macrophage inflammatory responses [59, 60]. On the other hand, it was found that bacterial DNA enhances expression of CD11b genes, while TLR9 expression in NG does not change under the influence of bacterial DNA [61].

Comparative evaluation of the effect of in vitro sodium deoxyribonucleate and the TLR9 agonist (ODN2395) on $CD16^{+}CD11b^{+}$subpopulation composition of NG in both healthy individuals and infectious diseases was of interest [62].

In particular, it was shown that when the peripheral blood of conventionally healthy volunteers with sodium deoxyribonucleate is incubated in vitro, the density of surface-localized CD11b and CD16 receptors is increased, which is expressed by a significant increase in the content of $CD16^{br}CD11b^{br}$NG. The effect of the TLR9 agonist (ODN2395) on this subpopulation in patients with AEBVI allowed us to identify a tendency to decrease its relative content, the effects of the TLR9 agonist and sodium deoxyribonucleate did not affect the relative content of $CD16^{br}CD11b^{br}$NH in patients with ABT (**Figures 4–6**).

The assessment of the content of the $CD16^{br}CD11b^{br}$NG subpopulation in the incubation of the peripheral blood of patients with acute viral and acute bacterial processes made it possible to reveal a significant immunomodulating effect only in the experiment with sodium deoxyribonucleate. When the blood of patients with AEBVI was incubated, a significant decrease in the initially high relative content of $CD16^{br}CD11b^{br}$NG was found.

In acute bacterial infection (ABT), there was an increase in the percentage of $CD16^{br}CD11b^{dim}$NG and a decrease in the initially predominant subpopulation of $CD16^{dim}CD11b^{dim}$NG (as in incubation with sodium deoxyribonucleate and with the TLR9 agonist), whereas in acute EBV infection, an increase in $CD16^{br}CD11b^{dim}$NG was observed under the influence of sodium deoxyribonucleate in vitro (**Figure 4**).

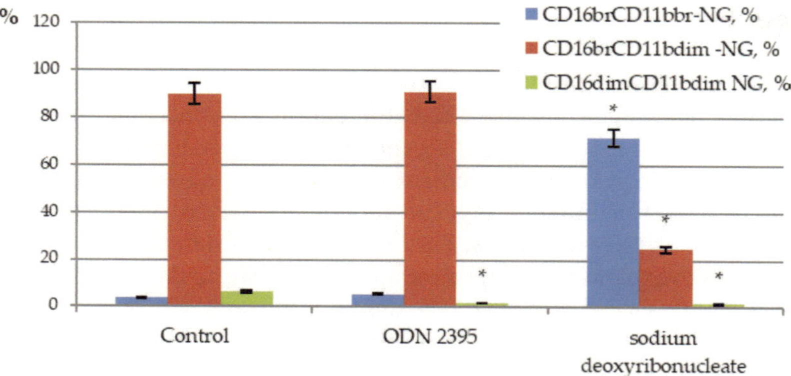

Figure 4.
Comparative analysis of the effect of the TLR9 agonist and sodium deoxyribonucleate in vitro on the subpopulation of $CD16^{+}CD11b^{+}$NG of healthy volunteers.

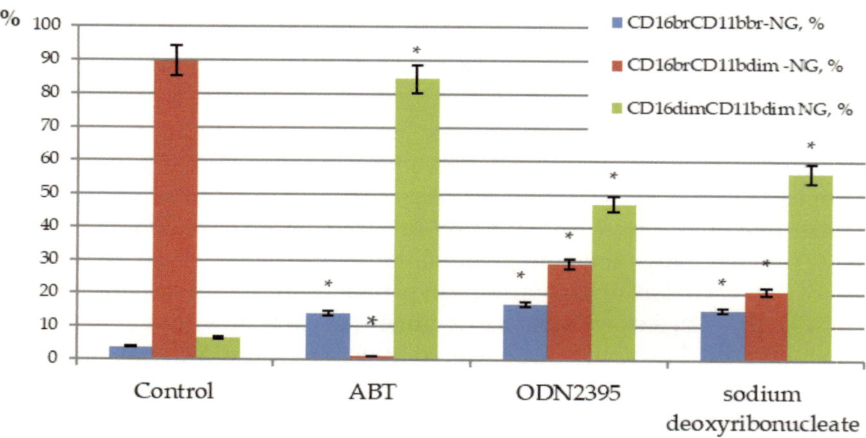

Figure 5.
Comparative analysis of the effect of the TLR9 agonist and sodium deoxyribonucleate in vitro on the subpopulation composition of $CD16^{+}CD11b^{+}$NG in patients with ABT.

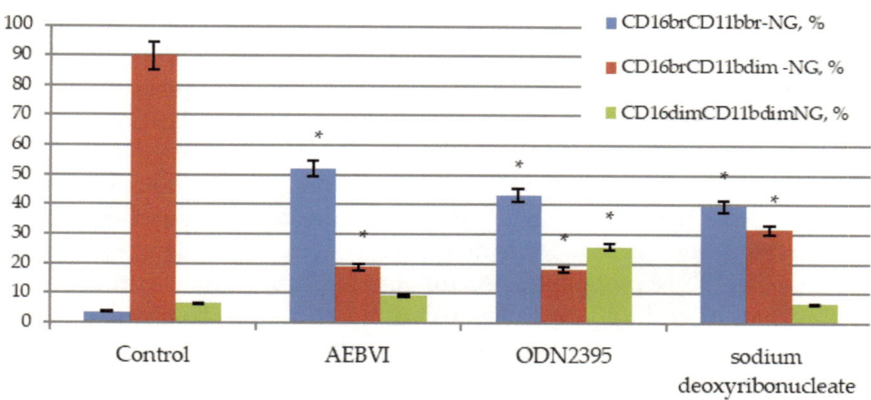

Figure 6.
Comparative analysis of the effect of the TLR9 agonist and sodium deoxyribonucleate in vitro on the subpopulation of $CD16^{+}CD11b^{+}$NG in patients with acute EBV infection.

It is important to note that the redistribution of NG subpopulation composition occurring under the action of both agonist and, especially, sodium deoxyribonucleate has a modulating nature, which suggests the involvement of Toll-like type 9 receptors in the regulation of functional NG activity in infectious processes.

5. Conclusion

The classical view of the NG, as short-lived finally differentiated cells, which carry out only phagocytosis, killing, and elimination of extracellular pathogens, is convincingly refuted by numerous recent studies. New scientific facts obtained during the last 10–15 years have demonstrated that NGs possess certain regulatory influences of activating, modulating, and suppressive nature, practically on all cells, both innate and adaptive immunity. The development of new diagnostic technologies allowed us to expand and deepen our understanding of the role of the NG in immune homeostasis and to evaluate the dynamic interrelation of the functional potential of the cell with gene expression and phenotypic polarization of the NG in response to inducing signals of intra- and extracellular environment. It is important to note that, to date, not all NG subpopulations have been identified.

Today it is well known that the population of $CD16^{+}CD11b^{+}$NG plays an important role in the reactions of phagocytosis and ADCC in infectious processes of various natures. It is also known that CD11b and CD16 NG are the most important triggers inducing the cascade of activation and regulatory processes of the NG. The resting unactivated NGs express the low levels of CD11b and CD16 membrane molecules. After activation additional translocation of intracellular CD16 and CD11b molecules to the NG membrane takes place [6, 36, 63]. Our studies showed that the subpopulation $CD16^{bright}CD11b^{dim}$NG prevailed in healthy people, and the NG with the phenotype $CD16^{bright}CD11b^{bright}$ was absent in healthy volunteers but appeared and dominated in patients with acute EBV infection. It has been established that $CD16^{bright}CD11b^{dim}$NG subpopulation predominates in healthy individuals, subpopulation $CD16^{bright}CD11b^{bright}$NG prevails in patients with acute viral infection, and $CD16^{dim}CD11b^{bright}$NG subpopulation dominates in patients with acute bacterial infection. Identified by us in acute bacterial infection (acute bacterial tonsillitis), emergence of the prevalent population of $CD16^{dim}CD11b^{bright}$ NG indicated, in our opinion, the release into circulation of immature forms of NG in a bacterial attack. At the same time, $CD16^{bright}CD11b^{bright}$ NG subpopulation predominated in patients with acute viral infection (acute EBV infection). We hypothesized that on the one hand, the appearance of $CD16^{bright}CD11b^{bright}$ NG with high cytotoxicity (high levels of CD16 expression) and with a suppressive effect on T-cell proliferation (high levels of CD11b molecules) is necessary for the implementation of antiviral activity of the NG in their fight against EBV infection. $CD16^{bright}CD11b^{bright}$NG should have high antiviral activity. On the other hand, their suppressor properties (high levels of CD11b expression) may lead to various complications in the form of secondary bacterial infections. Thus, in severe acute EBV infection, we revealed the transformation of the NG phenotype and the appearance of a new subpopulation of $CD16^{bright}CD11b^{bright}$NG with high cytotoxicity and suppressive effects. Further studies are needed to determine the functional significance of the $CD16^{bright}CD11b^{bright}$ NG subpopulation for both EBV infection and other herpesvirus infections. In addition, early diagnosis of the etiological factors that cause an acute infectious process of a viral or bacterial nature is extremely important for the appointment of early etiopathogenetic therapy. The results of the present study demonstrate that the determination of various subpopulations of the NG in the early stages of an acute infectious process can contribute to the early differentiation of an acute viral process in which the $CD16^{bright}CD11b^{bright}$ NG subpopulation dominates and the acute bacterial process dominated by the $CD16^{dim}CD11b^{bright}$ NG subpopulation. On the other hand, it is extremely important to search for new substances that have immunomodulatory effects on the "negatively transformed" phenotype of the NG with the possibility of positive remodeling, which can prevent the attachment of serious complications, both in viral and bacterial infections [63].

Our studies of the eukaryotic DNA sodium salt effect on the expression of functionally significant CD16 and CD11b NG receptors in healthy individuals and in infectious diseases of viral and bacterial etiology have demonstrated the potential for transformation of the negatively altered phenotype of the NG, in particular, by remodeling the expression of CD11b on the NG membrane [64]. The obtained data open certain prospects for the development of new therapeutic strategies that allow correcting the negatively transformed phenotype of various subpopulations of defective functioning NG in severe infectious and inflammatory processes, both viral and bacterial etiologies.

Conflict of interest

Authors declare that there is no conflict of interest.

Author details

Irina V. Nesterova*, Galina A. Chudilova, Svetlana V. Kovaleva,
Lyudmila V. Lomtatidze and Tatyana V. Rusinova
Kuban State Medical University, Krasnodar, Russia

*Address all correspondence to: inesterova1@yandex.ru

References

[1] Bux J. Nomenclature of granulocyte antigens. Transfusion. 1999;**39**:662-663

[2] Fuchs T, Püellmann K, Scharfenstein O, Eichner R, Stobe E, Becker A, et al. The neutrophil recombinatorial TCR-like immune receptor is expressed across the entire human life span but repertoire diversity declines in old age. Biochemical and Biophysical Research Communications. 2012;**419**(2):309-315

[3] Matzinger P. Friendly and dangerous signals: Is the tissue control? Nature Immunology. 2007;**8**:11-13

[4] Cassatella MA. On the production of TNF-related apoptosis inducing ligand (TRAIL/Apo-2L) by human neutrophils. Journal of Leukocyte Biology. 2006;**79**:1140-1149

[5] Kiseleva EP. New ideas about anti-infectious immunity. Infection and Immunity. 2011;**1**(1):9-14

[6] Elghetany MT. Surface antigen changes during normal neutrophilic development: A critical review. Blood Cells, Molecules & Diseases. 2002;**28**(2):260-274

[7] Nesterova IV, Kovaleva SV, Evglevsky AA, Chudilova GA, Lomtididze LV, Fomicheva EV. Remodeling of chromatin structure and change of the phenotype of neutrophilic granulocytes under the influence of G-CSF in patients with colorectal cancer. Modern Problems of Science and Education. 2014;**3**:1-8. http://science-education.ru/ru/article/view?id=13006

[8] Nesterova IV, Kolesnikova NV, Kleshchenko EI, Tarakanov VA, Smerchinskaya TV, Sapun OI, et al. Different variants of defects in the functioning of neutrophilic granulocytes in congenital pneumonia in newborns. Russian Immunological Journal. 2012;**6**(2):170-176

[9] Beyrau M, Bodkin JV, Nourshargh S. Neutrophil heterogeneity in health and disease: A revitalized avenue in inflammation and immunity. Open Biology. 2012;**2**(11):120-134

[10] Nesterova IV, Kovaleva SV, Chudilova GA, Lomatidze LV, Yevlevsky AA. The dual role of neutrophilic granulocytes in the implementation of antitumor protection. Immunology. 2012;**33**(5):281-288

[11] Pillay J, Kamp VM, van Hoffen E, Visser T, Tak T, Lammers JW, et al. Subset of neutrophils in human systemic inflammation inhibits T cell responses through Mac-1. The Journal of Clinical Investigation. 2012;**122**(1):327-336

[12] Matsushima H, Geng S, Lu R, Okamoto T, Yao Y, Mayuzumi N, et al. Neutrophil differentiation into a unique hybrid population exhibiting dual phenotype and functionality of neutrophils and dendritic cells. Blood. 2013;**121**(10):1677-1689

[13] Nesterova IV, Kolesnikova NV, Chudilova GA, Lomatidze LV, Kovaleva SV, Yevlevsky AA. Neutrophilic granulocytes: A new look at the "old players" on the immunological field. Immunology. 2015;**35**(4):257-265

[14] Metelitsa LS, Gillies SD, Super M, Shimada H, Reynolds CP, Seeger RC. Antidisialoganglioside/granulocyte macrophage—colony-stimulating factor fusion protein facilitates neutrophil antibody-dependent cellular cytotoxicity and depends on FcγRII (CD32) and Mac-1 (CD11b/CD18) for enhanced effector cell adhesion and azurophil granule exocytosis. Blood. 2002;**99**(11):4166-4173

[15] Nesterova IV, Kolesnikova NV, Kleshchenko EI, Chudilova GA, Lomtididze LV, Smerchinskaya TV, et al. Variants of the transformation of the phenotype of neutrophilic granulocytes CD64+CD32+CD11b+ in newborns with various infectious and inflammatory diseases. Cytokines and Inflammation. 2011;**10**(4):61-65

[16] Nesterova IV, Kovaleva SV, Chudilova GA, Kokov EA, Lomtatidze LV, Storozhuk SV, et al. Peculiarities of the phenotype of neutrophilic granulocytes in neoplastic processes. Russian Immunological Journal. 2010;**4**(4(13)):374-380

[17] Kolesnikova NV, Kovaleva SV, Nesterova IV, Chudilova GA, Lomtatidze LV. Correction of violations of receptor function of neutrophilic granulocytes at the stage of pregravid preparation. Russian Immunological Journal. 2014;**8**(3(17)):697-699

[18] Nesterova IV, Chudilova GA, Lomatidze LV, Kovaleva SV, Sapun OI, Kleshchenko EI, et al. Remodeling of the phenotype of CD64-CD16+CD32+CD11b+ and CD64+CD16+CD32+CD11b+ neutrophilic granulocyte subspecies in congenital pneumonia in deeply premature neonates. Russian Journal of Immunology. 2014;**8**(17):1, 48-53

[19] Nesterova IV, Kovaleva SV, Kolesnikova NV, Kleshchenko EI, Shinkareva ON, Chudilova GA, et al. Optimization of interferon-and immunotherapy in immunocompromised children with associated viral infections. In: Allergy, Asthma & Immunophysiology: From basic science to clinical management. Medimond. International Proceedings. 2013. pp. 101-104

[20] Cortjens B, Ingelse SA, Calis JC, Valar AP, Koendetman L, Bem RA, et al. Neutrophil subset responses in infants with severe viral respiratory infection. Clinical Immunology. 2017;**176**:100-106

[21] Lukens MV, van de Pol AC, Coenjaerts FE, Jansen NJ, Kamp VM, Kimpen JL, et al. A systemic neutrophil response precedes robust CD8(+) T-cell activation during natural respiratory syncytial virus infection in infants. Journal of Virology. 2010;**84**(5):2374-2383

[22] Scapini P, Cassatella MA. Social networking of human neutrophils within the immune system. Blood. 2014;**124**(5):710-719

[23] Leliefeld PH, Wessels CM, Leenen LP, Koenderman L, Pillay J. The role of neutrophils in immune dysfunction during severe inflammation. Critical Care. 2016;**20**:73

[24] Pillay J, Tak T, Kamp VM, Koenderman L. Immune suppression by neutrophils and granulocytic myeloid-derived suppressor cells: Similarities and differences. Cellular and Molecular Life Sciences. 2013;**70**(20):3813-3827

[25] Woodfin AL, Voisin MB, Beyrau M, Colom B, Caille D, Diapouli FM, et al. The junctional adhesion molecule JAM-C regulates polarized transendothelial migration of neutrophils in vivo. Nature Immunology. 2011;**12**(8):761-769

[26] De Oliveira-Junior EB, Bustamante J, Newburger PE, Condino-Neto A. The human NADPH oxidase: Primary and secondary defects impairing the respiratory burst function and the microbicidal ability of phagocytes. Scandinavian Journal of Immunology. 2011;**73**(5):420-427

[27] Klebanoff SJ, Kettle AJ, Rosen H, Winterbourn CC, Nauseef WM. Myeloperoxidase: A front-line defender against phagocytosed

microorganisms. Journal of Leukocyte Biology. 2013;**93**(2):185-198

[28] Winterbourn CC, Kettle AJ. Redox reactions and microbial killing in the neutrophil phagosome. Antioxidants & Redox Signaling. 2013;**18**(6):642-660

[29] Markova TP. Often Ill Children. The Look of the Immunologist. Moscow: Torus Press; 2014. 192 p

[30] Khaitov RM, Ignatieva GA, Sidorovich IG. Immunology. Norm and Pathology. 3rd ed. Moscow: Medicine; 2010. 752p

[31] Wynn JL, Levy O. Role of innate host defenses in susceptibility to early-onset neonatal sepsis. Clinics in Perinatology. 2010;**37**(2):307-337

[32] Maródi L. Innate cellular immune responses in newborns. Clinical Immunology. 2006;**118**(2-3):137-144

[33] Drifte G, Dunn-Siegrist I, Tissières P, Pugin J. Innate immune functions of immature neutrophils in patients with sepsis and severe systemic inflammatory response syndrome. Critical Care Medicine. 2013;**41**(3):820-832

[34] Oku R, Oda S, Nakada TA, Sadahiro T, Nakamura M, Hirayama Y, et al. Differential pattern of cell-surface and soluble TREM-1 between sepsis and SIRS. Cytokine. 2013;**61**(1):112-117

[35] Gusakova NV, Novikova IA. Functional activity of neutrophils in chronic recurrent herpetic infection. Medical Immunology. 2013;**15**(2):169-176

[36] Rusinova TV, Chudilova GA, Kolesnikova NV. Comparative evaluation of immunotropic effects in vitro of derinata and synthetic agonist TLR9 on the receptor function of neutrophilic granulocytes and monocytes in normal and in infectious process. Kuban Scientific Medical Journal. 2016;**5**(160):94-97

[37] Pillay J, den Braber I, Vrisekoop N, Kwast LM, de Boer RJ, Borghans JA, et al. In vivo labeling with 2H2O reveals a human neutrophil lifespan of 5.4 days. Blood. 2010;**116**(4):625-627

[38] Zlotnikova MV, Novikova IA. Functional activity of neutrophils and peroxidation of lipids in severe form of herpetic infection. Problems of Health and Ecology. 2011;**27**(1):70-76

[39] Didkovskii NA, Malashenkova IK, Tanasova AN, Shepetkova IN, Zuikov IA. Herpesvirus infection: The clinical significance and principles of therapy. BC. 2004;**12**(7):459-464

[40] Nagoev BS, Kambachokova ZA. Functional-metabolic activity of neutrophilic granulocytes in patients with recurrent herpetic infection. Journal of Infectology. 2011;**3**(3):38-41

[41] Novikova IA, Romanova OA. Features of the production of cytokines in recurrent herpetic infection. Medical Immunology. 2013;**15**(6):571-576

[42] Drescher B, Bai F. Neutrophil in viral infections, friend or foe? Virus Research. 2013;**171**:1:1-1:7

[43] Krause PJ, Malech HL, Kristie J, Kosciol CM, Herson VC, Eisenfeld L, et al. Polymorphonuclear leukocyte heterogeneity in neonates and adults. Blood. 1986;**68**:200-204

[44] Spiekermann K, Roesler J, Elsner J, Lohmann-Matthes ML, Welte K, Malech H, et al. Identification of the antigen recognized by the monoclonal antibody 31D8. Experimental Hematology. 1996;**24**:453-458

[45] Nesterova IV, Chudilova GA, Lomtatidze LV, Kovaleva SV,

Kolesnikova NV, Avdeeva MG, et al. Remodelling of the phenotype CD16⁺CD11b⁺ neutrophilic granulocytes granulocytes in acute Epstein-Barr viral infections. Allergy, asthma, COPD, immunophysiology & norehabilitology: Innovative technologies. In: Filodiritto International Proceedings; April; Bologna, Italy. 2017. pp. 181-187

[46] Elghetany MT, Lacombe F. Physiologic variations in granulocytic surface antigen expression: Impact of age, gender, pregnancy, race, and stress. Journal of Leukocyte Biology. 2004;**75**:157-162

[47] Pillay J, Ramakers BP, Kamp VM, Loi ALT, Lam SW, Falco H, et al. Functional heterogeneity and differential priming of circulating neutrophils in human experimental endotoxemia. Journal of Leukocyte Biology. 2010;**88**(1):211-220

[48] Kushner BH, Cheung NK. Absolute requirement of CD11/CD18 adhesion molecules, FcRII and the phosphatidylinositollinked FcRIII for monoclonal antibody-mediated neutrophil antihuman tumor cytotoxicity. Blood. 1992;**79**(6):1484-1490

[49] Filatov OY, Kashaeva OV, Bugrimov DY, Klimovich AA. Morphophysiological principles of immunological action of eukaryotic DNA. Russian Immunological Journal. 2013;7(16):4

[50] Rykova EY, Laktionov PP, Vlasov VV. Activating influence of DNA on the immune system. Advances of Modern Biology. 2001;**121**(2):160-171

[51] Besednova NN, Zaporozhets TS. The action of deoxyribonucleic acid prokaryotes on the humoral and cellular factors of congenital and adaptive immunity of vertebrates. Pacific Medical Journal. 2009;**3**:8-12

[52] Shutikova AN, Zaporozhets TS, Serebryakova MF, Epstein LM, Korneeva NA. The effect of DNAC on immunity indices in elderly people. Journal of Microbiology, Epidemiology and Immunobiology. 2006;**3**:68-71

[53] Goldfarb Y, Levi B, Sorski L, Frenkel D, Ben-Eliyahu S. CpG-C immunotherapeutic efficacy is jeopardized by ongoing exposure to stress: Potential implications for clinical use. Brain, Behavior, and Immunity. 2011;**25**:67-76

[54] Takeda K, Sh A. Toll-like receptors in innate immunity. International Immunology. 2005;**17**:1:1-1:14

[55] Berezhnaya NM, Sepiashvili RI. Physiology of TOLL-like receptors—Regulators of congenital and acquired immunity. Journal of Physiology. 2011;**57**(5):26-29

[56] Hyang LT, Paredes CG, Papoutsakis ET, Miller WM. Gene expression analysis illuminates the transcriptional programs underlying the functional activity of ex vivo-expanded granulocytes. Physiological Genomics. 2007;**31**(10):114-125

[57] Yoshimura A, Ohishi HM, Aki D, Hanada T. Regulation of TLR signaling and inflammation by SOCS family proteins. Journal of Leukocyte Biology. 2004;**5**(3):422-427

[58] Figueiredo MM. Expression of Toll–like receptors 2 and 9 in cells of dog jejunum and colon naturally infected with leishmania infantum. BMC Immunology. 2013;**14**(22):1-12. http://www.biomedcentral.com/1471-2172/14/22

[59] Bai Y. Integrin CD11b negatively regulates TLR9–triggered dendritic cell cross–priming by upregulating microRNA–146a. The Journal of Immunology. 2012;**188**(11):5293-5302

[60] Han C. Integrin CD11b negatively regulates TLR–triggered inflammatory responses by activating Syk and promoting degradation of MyD88 and TRIF via Cbl–b. Nature Immunology. 2010;**11**:734-742

[61] Itagaki K, Adibnia Y, Sun S. Bacterial DNA induces pulmonary damage via TLR9 through cross–talk with neutrophils. Shock. 2011;**36**(6):548-552

[62] Rusinova TV, Kolesnikova NV, Chudilova GA, et al. Comparative evaluation of the immunotropic effects of TLR9 agonists and the sodium salt of vertebrate DNA in normal and infectious processes. Russian Immunological Journal. 2016;**10/2**(19/1):77-79

[63] Nesterova IV, Chudilova GA, Lomtatidze LV, Kovaleva SV, Kolesnikova NV, Avdeeva MG, et al. Differentiation of variants of subpopulations of the transformed CD16+CD11b+ phenotype of neutrophilic granulocytes in acute viral and acute bacterial infections. Immunology. 2016;**37**(4):199-204

[64] Tamassia N, Cassatella MA, Bazzoni F. Fast and accurate quantitative analysis of cytokine gene expression in human neutrophils. Methods in Molecular Biology. 2014;**1124**:451-467

Chapter 5

Essence of Reducing Equivalent Transfer Powering Neutrophil Oxidative Microbicidal Action and Chemiluminescence

Robert C. Allen

Abstract

Neutrophil leukocytes provide first-line phagocytic defense against infection. Phagocyte locomotion to the site of infection, identification, and phagocytosis of the infecting microbe results in metabolically driven O_2-dependent combustive microbicidal action. NADPH oxidase activity controls this respiratory burst metabolism. Its flavoenzyme character allows semiquinone-mediated crossover from two reducing equivalents (2RE) to 1RE transfer, as is necessary for univalent reduction of O_2 to the acid hydroperoxyl radical (HO_2) and its conjugate base, superoxide anion (O_2^-). RE transfer dynamics is considered from the perspectives of quantum and particle physics, as well as frontier orbital interactions. Direct disproportionation of HO_2-O_2^- yields electronically excited singlet molecular oxygen ($^1O_2^*$) and hydrogen peroxide (H_2O_2). Myeloperoxidase catalyzes H_2O_2-dependent 2RE oxidation of chloride (Cl^-) to hypochlorite (OCl^-). Direct nonenzymatic reaction of OCl^- with an additional H_2O_2 yields Cl^-, H_2O, and $^1O_2^*$. Thus, for two 2RE metabolized through NADPH oxidase, a total of three $^1O_2^*$ are possible. H_2O_2, OCl^-, and $^1O_2^*$ generated are all singlet multiplicity reactants and can participate in spin-allowed combustive oxygenations yielding light emission, that is, luminescence or chemiluminescence. The sensitivity of luminescence for measuring neutrophil redox activities is increased several orders of magnitude by introducing chemiluminigenic probes. Probes can be selected to differentiate oxidase from haloperoxidase activities.

Keywords: neutrophil, respiratory burst, reducing equivalent, combustion, frontier orbital, spin quantum number, NADPH oxidase, myeloperoxidase, Wigner spin conservation, Hund's maximum multiplicity rule, boson, fermion

1. Introduction

> *There is a complicated hypothesis, which usually entails an element of mystery and several unnecessary assumptions. This is opposed by a more simple explanation, which contains no unnecessary assumptions. The complicated one is always the popular one at first, but the simpler one, as a rule, eventually is found to be correct. This process*

> *frequently requires 10–20 years. The reason for this long time lag was explained by Max Planck. He remarked that scientists never change their minds, but eventually they die.*
>
> John H. Northrop, 1961 [1].

Appreciating why combustion is not spontaneous, how electrons are transferred biologically, and the unusual nature of oxygen reactivity were difficult for me as a student. So, in addition to biochemical studies, my mentor Richard Steele suggested I study the writings of Herzberg and others. Although challenging, such exposure shook open the door to other perspectives. Fundamental quantum and particle physics considerations were entertained with regard to oxygen and biologic electron transfer. My epiphany was in recognizing that the polymorphonuclear neutrophil, a leukocyte familiar to me from clinical laboratory experience, might realize the electronegative potential of oxygen for combustive microbicidal action by changing the spin multiplicity of oxygen. The following, taken from a symposium abstract presented in 1972, succinctly describes that position [2]. "Recently, a chemiluminescence (CL) has been observed when human polymorphonuclear leukocytes (PMN) phagocytize bacteria or particulate matter. The CL response correlates well with the stimulation of the hexose monophosphate shunt, which results in the generation of NADPH. The PMN possesses both CN^--insensitive NADH and NADPH oxidases. Flavoproteins oxidases of this type are capable of univalent reduction of O_2. The reduced oxygen ($\cdot O_2^-$, $\cdot O_2H$) may then disproportionate yielding HOOH and singlet molecular oxygen $^1O_2$. The PMN also possesses a CN^--sensitive peroxidase, myeloperoxidase, which has microbicidal activity in the presence of HOOH and halide. In this reaction, the HOOH is reduced to OH^- with the oxidation of the halide to a reactive halogonium species. In cases where the halogonium formed is Cl^+ or Br^+, there is potential for further reaction with HOOH resulting in the generation of a haloperoxy anion. This unstable species can disintegrate to yield the original halide and $^1O_2$. $^1O_2$ has been demonstrated to be a potent microbicidal agent. Therefore, the biochemical generation of $^1O_2$ by the PMN might be closely associated with microbicidal activity. The CL response may be the result of the relaxation of excited carbonyl groups generated via $^1O_2$-mediated oxidations."

Neutrophil leukocytes and monocytes play an essential role in innate phagocytic defense against infection. Immune surveillance mechanisms detect the presence of potentially pathologic microbes and generate the chemical signals that mobilize circulating neutrophils and prime the expression of receptors necessary for neutrophil navigation and phagocytosis. Contact of a primed neutrophil with activated endothelium is followed by neutrophil diapedesis into the tissue interstitial space, and locomotion to the site of infection guided by concentration gradients of complement anaphylatoxin, microbial products, cytokines, and lipid factors. Once an immunologically primed neutrophil contacts an opsonin-labeled pathogen, phagocytosis occurs. Phagocytosis is associated with a constellation of metabolic changes classically referred to as the "respiratory burst" [3]. This presentation focuses on the neutrophil redox mechanisms necessary for microbicidal action, especially the roles of NADPH oxidase and myeloperoxidase (MPO) in lethal microbicidal oxygenations. The Merriam-Webster dictionary defines combustion as a chemical reaction that occurs when oxygen combines with other substances to produce heat and usually light. By changing the spin multiplicity of oxygen from triplet to doublet, and then to singlet, neutrophils remove the spin barrier to direct oxygenation, enabling direct oxygen combustive microbicidal action with associated light emission, that is, chemiluminescence or luminescence [4].

2. Respiratory burst

The neutrophil "respiratory burst" describes the large increases in glucose consumption via the hexose monophosphate shunt (aka, pentose pathway) [5, 6], and in nonmitochondrial molecular oxygen (O_2) consumption [7] associated with phagocytosis, and required for microbicidal action. Appreciating the underlying necessity for such metabolic changes provides perception into oxygen chemistry and biochemistry, radical reactivity and combustion in general. The character of electron transfer mediated by the dehydrogenases of the hexose monophosphate (HMP) shunt is common to cytoplasmic redox reactions. Such oxidation-reduction transfers typically involve movement of two reducing equivalents (2RE), that is, 2 electrons (e^-) and 2 protons (H^+), from an organic substrate catalyzed by a dehydrogenase. In turn, the dehydrogenase mobilizes the 2RE by transfer to nicotinamide adenine dinucleotide (phosphate) $NAD(P)^+$ generating its reduced form NAD(P)H. The cofactors NADPH and NADH serve as the cytoplasmic redox carriers for 2RE transfers between dehydrogenases and oxidases, and are common to various pathways of cytoplasmic metabolism. Consumption of 2RE carried by NADPH returns it to $NADP^+$. Availability of $NADP^+$ is rate limiting for HMP shunt dehydrogenase activity. Dehydrogenation is a type of oxidation that does not require or directly involve O_2. Glucose-6-phosphate (G-6-P) dehydrogenase, the initiator enzyme of the HMP shunt removes a total of 2RE and transfers the 2RE to $NADP^+$ producing NADPH. The point for emphasis is that 2RE are transferred, not one. Such 2RE transfer, sometimes referred to as hydride ion (H^-) transfer, is the rule for cytoplasmic redox reactions [8].

Respiratory burst metabolism results from the activation of NADPH oxidase. Like many oxidases, NADPH oxidase is a flavoenzyme. Flavoenzymes are mechanistically unique in that 2RE reduction, by cofactors such as NAD(P)H, is followed by a series of 1RE oxidations. In its 1RE form, the riboflavin prosthetic group of flavin adenine dinucleotide (FAD) is in the semiquinone state [9, 10]. This semiquinone capability, usually in combination with a cytochrome component, allows the oxidase to transition from 2RE transfer to 1RE transfers. As such, flavoenzymes are the junction enzymes where 2RE transfer proceeds as 1RE cytochrome transfers, for example, the mitochondrial electron transport system or the microsomal cytochrome-P450 mixed-function oxidase system [10, 11]. Flavoprotein oxidases are also capable of catalyzing the 1RE reduction of O_2 [12, 13]. As such, phagocytosis-associated activation of NADPH oxidase opens the possibility for univalent, that is, 1RE, reduction of O_2.

The molecular oxygen we breathe has unique physical-chemical characteristics. In its ground, that is, lowest energy state, oxygen is a diradical, paramagnetic molecule with triplet spin multiplicity [$^3O_2$; the preceding superscripted (^{3}) indicates multiplicity]. These spin characteristics guarantee a tendency for $^3O_2$ to participate in 1RE reduction yielding the doublet multiplicity hydroperoxyl radical ($^2HO_2$) and its conjugate base, the superoxide anion radical ($^2O_2^-$) [2, 4, 14, 15]. Such reduction does not produce radical character; it decreases such character.

2.1 Bosonic character of coupled fermionic electron transfer

Movement of 2RE is the transfer of an electron couple, that is, an orbital pair of electrons. Such 2RE transfers are the rule in cytoplasmic redox reactions. Considered from the perspective of particle physics, movement of a single electron (1RE) is quite different from paired electron (2RE) movement. Transfer of 1RE is a fermionic transfer. An electron is a fermion, and fermions have wave functions that are antisymmetric to exchange of particles; that is, $\Psi(a, b) = -\Psi(b, a)$. Fermions anti-commute; that is, $a \times b \neq b \times a$. Rotating a fermion through 360°,

Ψ — 360° → $-\Psi$, changes the phase, but does not return the fermion to its original state. An additional 360° rotation, $-\Psi$ —360° → Ψ, is required to return the antisymmetric particle to its original state [16]. Fermions obey Fermi-Dirac statistics.

A fermionic electron is defined by its five quantum numbers: n, l, m_l, s, and m_s [17]. The spin number, s, describes the intrinsic angular momentum of the electron independent of orbital motion, and has a value of ½$\hbar$ (abbreviated to ½). This quality has no analogy in classical physics. The total spin angular momentum, S, of an atom or molecule is expressed by the equation $S = \sqrt{[s(s+1)]}\hbar$. s gives rise to the quantum number m_s, and only two values are allowed. When m_s = ½, the e^- is described as spin up (↑); when m_s = −½, the e^- is described as spin down (↓). The Pauli exclusion principle states that the total wave function for a system must be antisymmetric to the exchange of any pair of electrons. Differently stated, no two electrons of a given atom or molecule can have identical quantum numbers, and for two electrons to occupy an orbital, each electron must have opposite spins, that is, one orbital e^- must have an m_s = ½ (↑), the other orbital e^- must have an m_s = −½ (↓). Consequently, the total spin quantum number, S, for a filled orbital electron-couple is ½ + −½ = 0 (↑↓).

Bosons obey Bose-Einstein statistics, and have wave functions that are symmetric to exchange of a pair of particles; that is, $\Psi(a, b) = \Psi(b, a)$. They obey ordinary commutation, that is, $a \times b = b \times a$. Rotating a boson through 360°, Ψ — 360° → Ψ, returns it to its original state. Bosons, for example, photons are symmetric particles with integral spin. Likewise, a spin-balanced composite of fermionic particles, for example, an alpha particle with an S of 0, is bosonic. With regard to biochemical redox reactions, the coupling of antisymmetric fermions, for example, the coupled electrons of an orbital pair, result in a S = 0 state with bosonic symmetry. The transfer of 2RE describes the movement of a coupled electron pair with an S = 0 and is in essence a bosonic transfer.

2.2 Bosonic versus fermionic frontier orbital interactions

Chemistry is about the frontier orbital interactions of atoms and molecules [18]. The focus of frontier orbital theory is on the initial orbital conditions of the reactants and on reactive transition to product(s) with emphasis on the highest occupied atomic or molecular orbital (HO(A)MO) and the lowest unoccupied atomic or molecular (LU(A)MO) orbital. The frontier orbital of a radical reactant is neither empty nor completely filled, and as such, is described as a singly occupied atomic or molecular orbital (SOAO or SOMO). Atomic and molecular orbitals, including frontier orbitals, can have bosonic or fermionic character [19, 20]. A HO(A)MO has an S = 0. Such an atom or molecule has singlet spin multiplicity with nonradical, diamagnetic character. A radical SO(A)MO has an S = ½ or −½, and has doublet spin multiplicity with radical, paramagnetic character.

The bosonic character of the HOMO of a nonradical reactant differs fundamentally from the fermionic character of the SOMO of a radical reactant. The fermionic nature of a SOMA limits overlap possibilities with bosonic HOMO. If such reaction occurs, the fermionic character must be preserved in the product. The electronegative Fenton radical (^2OH) can extract 1RE from the HOMO of a singlet multiplicity nonradical substrate (^{1}substrate) yielding singlet multiplicity ^1H_2O, but in the process the HOMO of the substrate is converted to a SOMO, that is, the substrate becomes a doublet multiplicity radical (^{2}substrate). The symmetry of the reactants is preserved in the products. If a fermionic (doublet)-bosonic (singlet) reaction occurs, symmetry will be retained in the bosonic (singlet)-fermionic (doublet) products. Consistent with the Wigner-Witmer rules described in **Table 1**, spin symmetry is conserved [19–22].

The fermionic character of two radical reactants is eliminated in reactive bonding yielding a bosonic product. As described in **Table 1**, fermionic radical-radical, SOMO-SOMO reaction yields bosonic nonradical product. Simply stated, radicals

DOI: http://dx.doi.org/10.5772/intechopen.81543

tend to react with radicals, and such doublet-doublet annihilations yield nonradical, that is, bosonic, product. Such reaction is responsible for terminating radical chain propagation reactions.

Molecular oxygen in its ground state has unique triplet spin multiplicity [23]. Its two degenerate, that is, equal energy, frontier orbitals are each populated by a single electron. These two SOMO electrons obey Hund's maximum multiplicity rule, that is, the electron in each degenerate SOMO will have the same spin [24]. As illustrated in **Figure 1**, the ***S*** value for molecular oxygen is ½ + ½ or −½ + −½, and thus, the multiplicity is triplet, that is, 2|1 or −1| + 1 = 3. This bi-radical, bi-fermionic character is responsible for the paramagnetic character of $^3O_2$. The high electronegativity of $^3O_2$ predicts potential for highly exergonic reactions with nonradical, singlet multiplicity organic molecules, but thermodynamic potential does not guarantee reactivity, and combustion is not spontaneous. Taking a different perspective, it is

Reactants	Products
Singlet + Singlet bosonic + bosonic	Singlet bosonic
Singlet + Doublet bosonic + fermionic	Doublet fermionic
Singlet + Triplet bosonic + bi-fermionic	Triplet bi-fermionic
Doublet + Doublet fermionic + fermionic	Singlet bosonic
Doublet + Triplet fermionic + bi-fermionic	Doublet fermionic
Triplet + Triplet bi-fermionic + bi-fermionic	Singlet bosonic

Spin multiplicity states with regard to the bosonic-fermionic character of reactants and products.

Table 1.
Spin conservation rules.

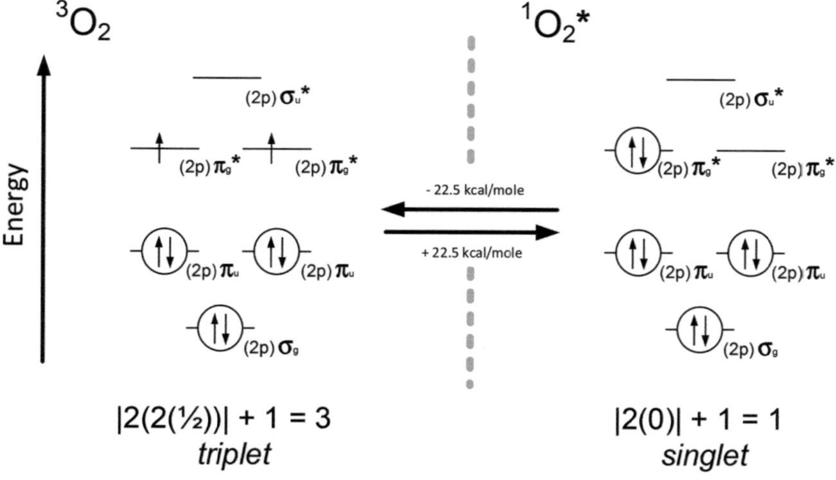

Figure 1.
Triplet and electronically excited singlet molecular oxygen with emphasis on the π (pi antibonding) frontier orbitals. The two π* are degenerate (same energy level). Hund's maximum multiplicity rule predicts lowest energy is achieved when each SOMO electron has the same spin, that is, the triplet state ($^3O_2$). The electronic energy of $^1O_2$* is 22.5 kcal/mol (94.2 kJ/mol) above $^3O_2$.*

the bi-fermionic, bi-radical nature of $^3O_2$ that restricts its reactive potential. As per **Table 1**, the reaction of $^3O_2$ with a bosonic ^{1}substrate molecules is spin symmetry restricted, and could only result in the improbable generation of a bi-fermionic, triplet multiplicity product(s). However, the reaction of bi-fermionic $^3O_2$ with a fermionic (doublet multiplicity) radical can proceed via SOMO-SOMO overlap. As per **Table 1**, such a doublet-triplet reaction will generate a fermionic (doublet multiplicity) radical product. Thus, $^3O_2$ can participate in and be a necessary reactant in radical propagation reactions.

3. NADPH oxidase

NADPH oxidase controls "respiratory burst" metabolism, microbicidal action, and chemiluminescence [15, 25]. The oxidase (Nox2) is a complex flavoenzyme, and a member of the Nox family of enzymes involved in various biochemical activities [26–29]. More specifically, NADPH oxidase is a flavocytochrome enzyme composed of a large membrane-bound glycoprotein ($gp91^{phox}$) subunit associated with a smaller protein ($p22^{phox}$). The C-terminal portion of $gp91^{phox}$ subunit contains the NADPH and flavin adenine dinucleotide (FAD) binding sites and an N-terminal portion that binds two heme groups. The activation of the oxidase is complex and involves other components. Association with the $p67^{phox}$ component is essential for full activity. The present treatment will focus on the central role of the semiquinone state of the riboflavin component of FAD and heme involvement in splitting the 2RE from ^{1}NADPH and facilitating 1RE reduction of $^3O_2$.

As illustrated in **Figure 2**, the product of 1RE reduction of $^3O_2$ is the acid hydroperoxyl radical ($^2HO_2$) with an acid dissociation constant pK_a of 4.8 [30]. For comparison, the pK_a of $^1H_2O_2$ is 11.7. As the pH of the phagolysosomal space approaches the pK_a, the ratio of $^2HO_2$ to its conjugate base, the superoxide anion ($^2O_2^-$) approaches unity, and acid disproportionation, that is, reaction of $^2HO_2$ with $^2O_2^-$, approaches maximum reaction rate. At unity, anionic repulsion is no longer a problem. The rate constant for the reaction is $4.5 \times 10^5\ M^{-1}\ s^{-1}$ at pH 7.0 and reaches a maximum of $8.5 \times 10^7\ M^{-1}\ s^{-1}$ at pH 4.8 [30, 31]. From the frontier orbital perspective, this is a SOMO-SOMO reaction that yields the nonradical (singlet multiplicity) products $^1H_2O_2$ and $^1O_2^*$. As per **Table 1**, doublet-doublet annihilation yields single products [15, 32]. The reaction is sufficiently exergonic to yield $^1O_2^*$ with an energy of 22.5 kcal/mol (94.1 kJ/mol) above ground state $^3O_2$.

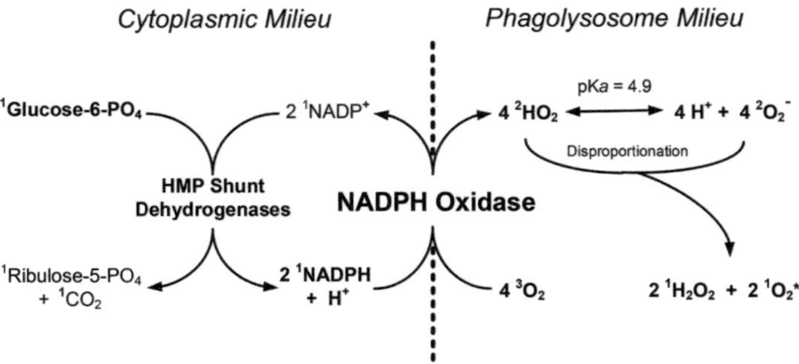

Figure 2.
Schema illustrating the central role of membrane-associated NADPH oxidase in respiratory burst metabolism. In the activated state, the Michaelis constant (K_M) of the oxidase for NADPH is decreased. $NADP^+$ availability controls the activities of glucose-6-PO_4 dehydrogenase and 6-phosphogluconate dehydrogenase of the HMP shunt. Each pass of the cycle generates two NADPH, that is, two 2RE. In the schema, the spin multiplicities of each molecule are indicated by the superscripted number preceding the molecular description, that is, ^{1}, ^{2}, and ^{3} for singlet, doublet, and triplet multiplicity, respectively.

In **Figure 2**, note that all reactions in the cytoplasmic milieu are singlet multiplicity nonradical reactions and that radical production is confined to the phagolysosomal milieu. The 2RE nature of cytoplasmic redox transfer provides a bosonic barrier to reaction with bi-fermionic $^3O_2$. Transfer of an orbital electron couple is nonradical, bosonic, and singlet multiplicity. In an atmosphere that is 20.9% $^3O_2$, the presence of a doublet multiplicity molecule is an opportunity for SOMO-SOMO overlap. The 2RE transfer from the HOMO of a reductant to the LUMO of an oxidant maintains the bosonic $\boldsymbol{S} = 0$ condition.

The $\boldsymbol{S} = 0$ condition is described by Dirac's statement that "If a state has zero total angular momentum, the dynamical system is equally likely to have any orientation, and hence spherical symmetry occurs" [33]. In addition to providing protection from the reactive consequences of fermionic 1RE transfer in an atmosphere high in $^3O_2$, 2RE transfer of a bosonic orbital electron couple may have additional advantage. Heisenberg's uncertainty principle states that the uncertainty of momentum (Δp) multiplied by the uncertainty of position (Δx) is always equal to or greater than ½$\hbar$, that is, $\Delta p \Delta x \geq \frac{1}{2}\hbar$ [17]. With regard to 2RE transfer, the bosonic orbital electron couple has $\boldsymbol{S} = 0$. Consequently, the positional uncertainty of the electron-couple must be proportionally large. The $\boldsymbol{S} = 0$ nature of HOMO-LUMO redox transfer involving a 2RE orbital electron-couple opens the possibility that such transfer is facilitated by quantum tunneling. The nature of such transfer would be analogous to the emission of a bosonic $\boldsymbol{S} = 0$ alpha particle from an atomic nucleus in alpha radiation decay [19, 20].

4. Myeloperoxidase

Myeloperoxidase (MPO) is a unique green cationic homo-dimeric glycosylated heme-a protein that is highly expressed in neutrophil leukocytes, making up about 5% of its dry mass [34, 35]. It is also synthesized to a lesser degree in monocytes and serves as a cellular marker for both neutrophils and monocytes. MPO synthesis occurs only during the promyelocyte phase of neutrophil development [36]. During the promyelocyte phase, MPO and other cationic lysosomal proteins are synthesized and stored in the azurophilic (aka primary) granules. Each mitotic division during the following myelocyte phase of development dilutes the azurophilic granule content per neutrophil by a half. Under normal conditions of hematopoietic production, these myelocytic phase mitoses are the rule, but under condition of neutrophil inflammatory consumption or G-CSF-stimulated marrow production, the promyelocyte pool is expanded, and there are fewer mitoses in the myelocyte phase of development. Neutrophils released into the circulation following a few days of myelopoietic stimulation show the effect of decreased myelocyte mitoses. These neutrophils are significantly increased in size due to greater azurophilic granule retention, and the MPO activity per neutrophil is severalfold higher than normal [37].

4.1 Electrochemistry of halide oxidation-reduction

MPO, like eosinophil peroxidase, lactoperoxidase and thyroperoxidase, is a haloperoxidase (XPO). However, MPO is unique in its ability to catalyze the pH-dependent oxidation of chloride [38–40]. Based on the Allen scale, fluorine (F) is the most electronegative element with a value of 4.19, followed by oxygen with a value of 3.61, then chlorine with a value of 2.87, bromine with a value of 2.69, and iodine with a value of 2.36 [41].

With regard to chloride oxidation, the Nernstian electrochemical possibilities and limitations are as follows [11, 42].

$$E = E_0 - (RT/nF)\ \ln\ [\text{reduced}]/[\text{oxidized}] \tag{1}$$

where E is observed potential (in volts), E_0 is the standard potential (in volts), R is the gas constant, T is the absolute temperature, F is a faraday (23 kcal/absolute volt equivalent), and n is the number of electrons/gram equivalent transferred.

Also, appreciate that hydrogen ion concentration, $[H^+]$, has an effect on redox chemistry.

$$E = (RT/F)\ \ln\ [H^+]/[P_{H2}]^{1/2} \tag{2}$$

P_{H2} is the partial pressure of H_2 gas

$$E = (2.3RT/F)\ \log\ [H^+] = 0.06\ \log\ [H^+] = -0.06\ pH \tag{3}$$

For the reaction, $A_{red} + B_{ox} \leftrightarrow B_{red} + D_{ox}$, the half reaction equations become:

$$E = E_0{}^{A} - (RT/nF)\ \ln\ [A_{red}]/[A_{ox}] \tag{4}$$

$$E = E_0{}^{B} - (RT/nF)\ \ln\ [B_{red}]/[B_{ox}] \tag{5}$$

$$E_0{}^{B} - E_0{}^{A} = (RT/nF)\ [\ln\ [B_{red}]/[B_{ox}] - \ln\ [A_{red}]/[A_{ox}]] \tag{6}$$

$$\Delta E_0 = (RT/nF)\ [\ln\ [A_{ox}][B_{red}]/\ln\ [A_{red}][B_{ox}]] \tag{7}$$

$$\Delta E_0 = (RT/nF)\ \ln K_{eq} \tag{8}$$

K_{eq} is the equilibrium constant. The change in potential (ΔE) can be expressed in terms of Gibbs free energy (ΔG).

$$\Delta G^0 = -RT \ln K_{eq} \tag{9}$$

$$\Delta G^0 = -nF\ \Delta E_0 \tag{10}$$

The schema of **Figure 3** depicts the MPO-catalyzed H_2O_2 oxidation of Cl^- to HOCl. Chloride serves as the reductant and undergoes a 2RE oxidization yielding a chloronium intermediate (Cl^+) that reacts with ^1H_2O to generate hypochlorous acid with a pKa of 7.5.

$$^1Cl^- \rightarrow {}^1Cl^+ + 2RE \tag{11}$$

$$^1Cl^+ + {}^1H_2O \rightarrow {}^1HOCl + H^+ \tag{12}$$

Note that $^1H_2O_2$ is the oxidant for the MPO-catalyzed reaction undergoing 2RE reduction yielding two waters. One ^1H_2O is consumed in the reaction described by Eq. (12).

$$^1H_2O_2 + 2RE \rightarrow 2\,^1H_2O \tag{13}$$

The reactants and products of this MPO-catalyzed redox reaction are exclusively singlet multiplicity, that is, nonradical [2, 15].

As depicted in **Figure 4**, increasing acidity, that is, lowering pH, increases the ΔE (i.e., $E_{H_2O_2} - E_{X^-}$) and the Gibbs free energy for all halides. The exergonicity of MPO-catalyzed 2RE dehydrogenation of Cl^- increases with increasing acidity. The required potentials for the various halides are consistent with their electronegativities. Dehydrogenation of Cl^- is more difficult than Br^-, but dehydrogenation of I^- is relatively easy. Whereas MPO is capable of dehydrogenating Cl^-, Br^-, and I^-, eosinophil peroxidase (EPO), lactoperoxidase, and thyroperoxidase are only capable of dehydrogenating Br^- and I^-.

The plots of **Figure 4** illustrate that increasing acidity increases the exergonicity of MPO-catalyzed $^1H_2O_2$-dependent oxidation of halides. This is especially import for MPO-catalyzed oxidation of chloride. Conversely, increasing alkalinity increases the exergonicity of the nonenzymatic $^1OCl^-$-$^1H_2O_2$ reaction yielding $^1O_2{}^*$ as depicted in **Figure 5**. The combined $^1H_2O_2$-driven haloperoxidase plus $^1H_2O_2$-driven $^1OCl^-$ generation of $^1O_2{}^*$ can be considered as a net disproportionation reaction, as depicted in **Figure 6**. $^1H_2O_2$ is the reactant common to both MPO-catalyzed reaction of **Figure 4** and the chemical reaction of **Figure 5**. The Gibbs free energies shown in

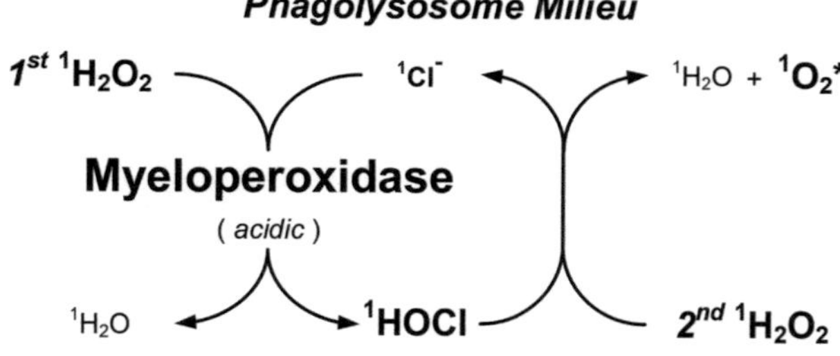

Figure 3.
Schema depicting myeloperoxidase-catalyzed H_2O_2-dependent oxidation of chloride to hypochlorite, and its reaction with a second H_2O_2 to generate $^1O_2{}^*$. The spin multiplicity of each molecule is indicated by the superscripted number preceding the molecular description.

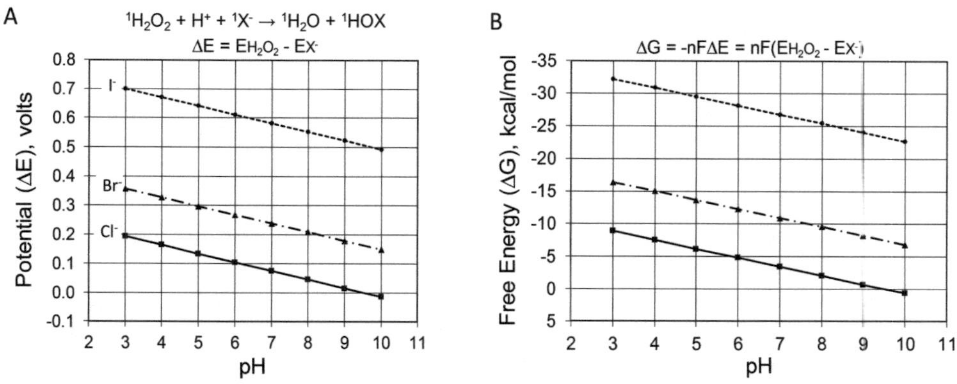

Figure 4.
*Graph **A** plots changes in potential (ΔE) and graph **B** plots change in Gibbs free energy against pH for various halides. From bottom to top, the plotted lines represent chloride (lowest), bromide (middle) and iodide (highest).*

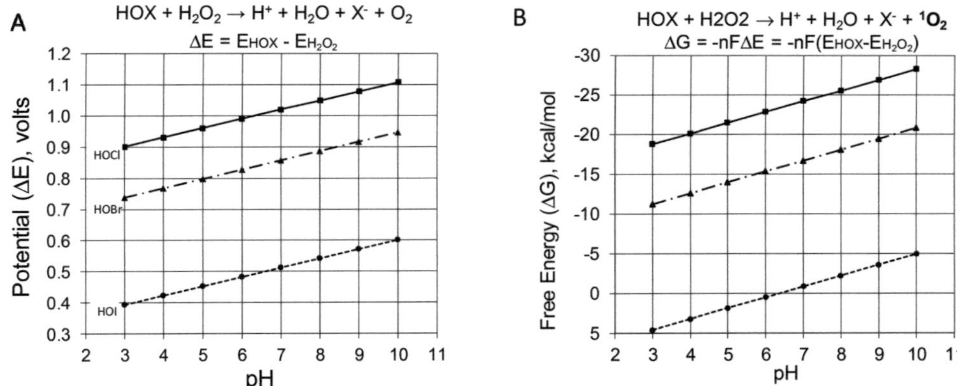

Figure 5.
*Graph **A** plots changes in potential (ΔE) and graph **B** plots change in Gibbs free energy with respect to pH for various halides for the reaction of $^1H_2O_2$ with $^1OCl^-$. In graph **B** the Gibbs free energies are adjusted for the 22.5 kcal mol^{-1} retained as the electronic energy of $^1O_2$*, that is, the difference separating $^3O_2$ from $^1O_3$*.*

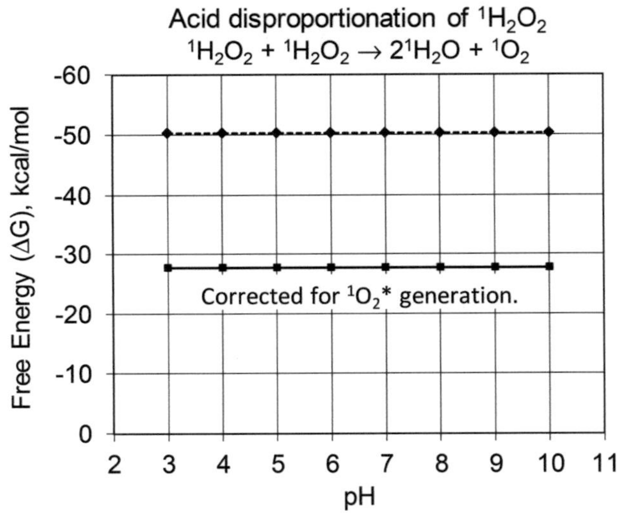

Figure 6.
*Plot of free energy against pH for the net $^1H_2O_2$ disproportionation reaction as described in **Figure 2**. The free energy results are expressed with ($\Delta G = -27.8$ kcal mol^{-1}) and without ($\Delta G = -50.3$ kcal mol^{-1}) adjustment for the energy electronically conserved in oxygen excitation ($\Delta G = -22.5$ kcal mol^{-1}).*

Figure 6 have been adjusted to reflect the energy conserved in electronically excited $^1O_2$*. The overall net free energy is independent of the halide employed and independent of pH.

Since the reactants involved are all singlet multiplicity, the products of reaction, that is, ^1H_2O, $^1Cl^-$, and $^1O_2$*, are all singlet multiplicity. This provides a spin symmetry explanation as to why pouring bleach ($^1OCl^-$) into $^1H_2O_2$ causes rapid reactive release of $^1O_2$* gas and a red chemiluminescence [23]. Caution, rapid release of gas is potentially explosive. When the concentration of $^1O_2$* is sufficiently high, $^1O_2$*-$^1O_2$* collision with simultaneous relaxation yields red chemiluminescence. The relaxation of one $^1O_2$* emits a 1270 nm photon; simultaneous relaxation of two $^1O_2$* emits a 635 nm photon. As such, this red emission is second order with respect to $^1O_2$*, that is, $dh\nu_{635nm}/dt = k[^1O_2^*]^2$, and is relatively short-lived.

The double dehydrogenation of ^{1}glucose-6-PO_4 produces ^{1}ribulose-5-PO_4 plus $^1CO_2$ plus two 2RE, that is, two bosonic electron couples carried as 2NADPH. As illustrated in **Figure 2**, NADPH oxidase reduces four $^3O_2$ in four one 1RE reduction steps, ultimately yielding two $^1O_2^*$ and two $^1H_2O_2$. As illustrated in **Figure 3**, MPO uses one $^1H_2O_2$ for oxidation of Cl^- to OCL^-, and this OCL^- reacts with the other $^1H_2O_2$ to generate an additional $^1O_2^*$. Thus, two NADPH have the potential to drive the generation of three $^1O_2^*$. Steinbeck et al. have reported experiments using glass beads coated with 9,10-diphenylanthracene, a $^1O_2^*$-specific trap, for measurements of neutrophil $^1O_2^*$ production [43]. Neutrophils were allowed to phagocytose the beads for an hour. The endoperoxide trapped indicated that at least 11.3 ± 4.9 nmol $^1O_2^*/1.25 \times 10^6$ neutrophils were produced. When the neutrophils were chemically activated with phorbol-12-myristate-13-acetate (PMA), at least 14.1 ± 4.1 nmol $^1O_2^*/1.25 \times 10^6$ neutrophils were produced. Based on their trapping results, $^1O_2^*$ production accounted for at least 19 ± 5% of the total oxygen consumed. Although the quantities of $^1O_2^*$ measured using this difficult trapping approach are lower than expected; this study provides direct empirical evidence of significant neutrophil $^1O_2^*$ production.

Quantifying cellular production of $^1O_2^*$ by measuring the 1270 nm near-infrared photon emitted on $^1O_2^*$ relaxation to $^3O_2$ is also problematic. Although highly specific for $^1O_2^*$, this infrared proton emission approach is highly insensitive in biological system measurements. The fact that a 1270 nm photon is measured is proof that $^1O_2^*$ did not participate in chemical reaction. Considering the variety of reactive substrates available in biological milieux, electrophilic reaction is favored over relaxation.

4.2 Myeloperoxidase-binding specificity focuses combustive activity

$^1O_2^*$ is a potent electrophilic reactant with a high probability for participation in spin-allowed reaction with electron-dense biological substrates. The lifetime of metastable electronically excited $^1O_2^*$ restricts its reactive possibilities [44]. In biological milieux, $^1O_2^*$ has a reactive lifetime of about 4–6 microseconds [45, 46]. This lifetime restricts reactivity to within a radius of about 0.2–0.3 μm (microns) from its point of generation. In the case of MPO generation of $^1O_2^*$, these temporal and spatial restrictions can be advantageous.

MPO selectively binds to all gram-negative bacteria and most gram-positive bacteria tested, but MPO binding is weak for gram-positive lactic acid bacteria (LAB) [44, 47]. LAB are common members of the normal flora of the mouth, vagina, and colon, and include streptococci, lactobacilli, and bifidobacteria. These LAB cannot synthesize cytochromes and produce lactic acid as a metabolic end product. They are typically microaerophilic, and often produce $^1H_2O_2$ as a metabolic product. The green hemolysis associated with colonies of viridans streptococci on blood agar plates results from the production of $^1H_2O_2$ by the streptococci. When a pathogen, such as *Staphylococcus aureus* or *Escherichia coli*, is contacted with a nonpathogen LAB, such as *Streptococcus viridans*, the pathogen overwhelmingly inhibits the LAB, but when a small quantity of MPO is added to a mixture, the pathogen is inhibited allowing LAB dominance. This phenomenon repeats even when erythrocytes are added to the mix at a ratio of 10 erythrocytes per bacteria. MPO selectively binds to the *S. aureus* and *E. coli* with essentially no binding to $^1H_2O_2$-producing *Strep. viridans*. Thus, LAB-produced $^1H_2O_2$ drives MPO microbicidal action that is restricted to the surface of the MPO-bound pathogen. MPO combustive microbicidal action is focused on the pathogen with minimum damage to the $^1H_2O_2$-producing LAB, and without hemolytic damage to the added erythrocytes, that is, no bystander injury.

Specificity of MPO binding results in specificity of microbicidal action. Binding specificity allows synergistic MPO-LAB interaction and suppression of pathogens. It also suggests a role for MPO in the selection and maintenance of LAB in the normal flora [48]. Healthy human adults release about a hundred billion MPO-rich neutrophils into the circulating blood each day. The circulating lifetime of the neutrophil is reportedly less than a day. The neutrophils then leave the blood and enter a tissue and body cavity phase lasting a few days [36]. Migration of MPO-rich neutrophils into the mouth and vagina is well-known [49, 50]. When quantified, the neutrophil count of the mouth is proportional to the blood neutrophil count. These spaces typically provide an acidic milieu. Neutrophil disintegration with MPO release may provide LAB with a selective advantage in such body spaces.

5. Microbicidal combustion and chemiluminescence

Reactions of ${}^1O_2^*$ with singlet multiplicity substrates (^{1}Sub) are spin-allowed and highly exergonic. The exergonicities of most biochemical reactions are sufficient for rotational and vibrational excitation, but not electronic excitation. Dioxygenation reactions are sufficiently exergonic for electronic excitation. Oxygenations producing singlet multiplicity endoperoxide and dioxetane intermediates are excellent candidates for luminescence [51]. The disintegrations of such intermediates generate $\mathbf{n\pi^*}$ electronically excited products, that is, an electron from the nonbonding (**n**) orbital of oxygen populates the pi antibonding ($\boldsymbol{\pi^*}$) orbital of the carbonyl. Singlet multiplicity $\mathbf{n\pi^*}$ excited molecules have short lifetimes. Electronic transition from the $\boldsymbol{\pi^*}$ of the carbonyl to the **n** of oxygen with photon emission is spin-allowed.

In addition to direct reaction of ${}^1O_2^*$ with ^{1}Sub, other singlet multiplicity reactants such as ${}^1OCl^-$ can react with ^{1}Sub to yield chloramine products (^{1}Sub-Cl) or dehydrogenated products (${}^1Sub_{-2RE}$). Such products can in turn react with ${}^1H_2O_2$ yielding endoperoxide or dioxetane intermediates with subsequent disintegration to $\mathbf{n\pi^*}$-excited carbonyl products relaxing by photon emission [52, 53]. The fundamental principle is that all reactants and products are singlet multiplicity nonradicals.

Dioxygenations yielding intermediate endoperoxide and dioxetanes disintegrate yielding an $\mathbf{n\pi^*}$ electronically excited carbonyl. **Figure 7** illustrates the energy and orbital differences that characterize the carbonyl states. Physical generation of a $\mathbf{n\pi^*}$ electronically excited carbonyl occurs when a fluorescent compound in its ground state absorbs a photon of appropriate energy. Because the ground state of the carbonyl is singlet, an electronically excited singlet multiplicity carbonyl undergoes rapid spin-allowed relaxation to ground state with a lifetime of less than 10^{-8} second [51]. Fluorescence describes photon-generated excitation followed by photon emission. Chemiluminescence or luminescence describes chemically generated electronic excitation followed by photon emission.

The metabolic changes of the respiratory burst describe the movement of RE required to change the spin multiplicity of ${}^3O_2$ from triplet to doublet (${}^2HO_2$), and ultimately to singlet, that is, ${}^1H_2O_2$ and ${}^1O_2^*$. MPO catalyzes the 2RE oxidation of ${}^1Cl^-$ to ${}^1HOCl$ followed by chemical reaction with a second ${}^1H_2O_2$ to generate ${}^1O_2^*$. Changing the bi-fermionic ${}^3O_2$ to bosonic ${}^1O_2^*$eliminates the spin barrier to direct dioxygenation of bosonic singlet multiplicity biological molecules. If intermediate endoperoxides and dioxetanes are generated, their disintegration yields electronically excited $\mathbf{n\pi^*}$ carbonyl functions that relax by photon emission. By changing the spin multiplicity of oxygen, neutrophil leukocytes realize its electronegative potential for combustive microbicidal action. Such combustion generates electronically excited products emitting light in the visible range of the spectrum.

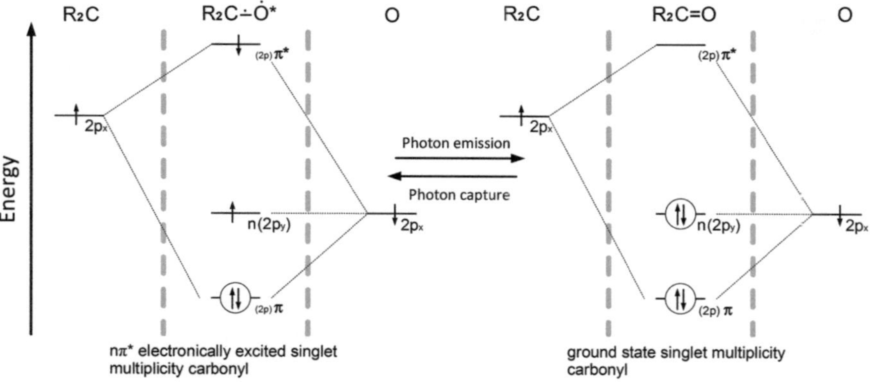

Figure 7.
Orbital diagram plot depicting the **nπ*** *electronically excited singlet state and the singlet ground state of a carbonyl. The gray dashed brackets indicate the carbonyl with the participating carbon and oxygen atoms shown on to the left and right, respectively. In the carbonyl diagram on the left, the* **nπ*** *notation indicates that an electron of the nonbonding (***n***) orbital of the carbonyl oxygen atom has been excited to the pi antibonding (π*) orbital of the carbonyl. Although excited, the electrons remained paired and the excited state is singlet multiplicity. Electron relaxation from* **π***-to-**n** *yields photon emission.*

6. Chemiluminigenic probes

The native chemiluminescence of neutrophils is proportional to respiratory burst activity [4, 54]. Since the luminescence resulting from microbicidal combustion is proportional to dioxygenations, especially those yielding endoperoxide and dioxetane intermediates, it follows that native neutrophil luminescence is influenced by the molecular composition of the microbe combusted. Native luminescence from phagocytosing neutrophils can be detected using less than a million neutrophils. For perspective, a milliliter of normal human blood contains about 4 million neutrophils. The native luminescence product of neutrophil combustive action is of low intensity. However, electronic excitation and the resultant luminescence is unambiguous evidence of neutrophil combustive dioxygenation action. Native luminescence has been usefully applied to measurement of neutrophil metabolic defects, e.g., chronic granulomatous disease [54, 55], and neutrophil responsiveness to humoral immune factors, such as complement and immunoglobulins [56].

Inclusion of high quantum yield chemiluminigenic substrates as probes (CLP) of neutrophil dioxygenation activities greatly increases the sensitivity and, to some degree, the specificity for detecting such activities [52, 57, 58]. With regard to increasing sensitivity, a CLP must be susceptible to neutrophil dioxygenation activities. This is achieved when endoperoxide or dioxetane intermediate are produced. The breakdown of such intermediates yields electronically excited **nπ*** carbonyl functions that relax by light emission. Use of a CLP typically increases the sensitivity for detecting dioxygenation activity by several orders of magnitude. Selecting a CLP with reactive specificity also provides information with regard to the nature of neutrophil activity measured.

6.1 Probing reductive oxygenation activity with lucigenin

Phagocytic or chemical activation of neutrophil respiratory burst metabolism can be tested using the dye nitro-blue tetrazolium (NBT) [59]. The NBT reaction measures neutrophil reduction activity, not neutrophil oxidation activity. A positive NBT result requires neutrophil respiratory burst activity resulting in reduction of the tetrazolium ring of the dye to a dark blue water-insoluble formazan precipitate. NBT is a large complex nitrogen heterocyclic compound with abundant resonance and electron delocalization possibilities. That NBT reduction might be linked to neutrophil univalent reduction of molecular oxygen was considered, and we observed that adding a small grain of potassium superoxide (KO_2) to a solution of NBT resulted in immediate reduction of the dye to a dark blue formazan precipitate [15]. Normal neutrophils reduce NBT upon activation of NADPH oxidase. The neutrophils of chronic granulomatous disease patients have defective NADPH oxidase, and as such, are incapable of NBT reduction [60].

Lucigenin (aka, bis-*N*-methylacridinium nitrate, or dimethyl biacridinium nitrate ($^1DBA^{+2}$)) is a heterocyclic organic compound known to generate chemiluminescence as a product of base-catalyzed peroxidation [61]. If sufficiently alkaline, singlet multiplicity ^{1}lucigenin reacts with the conjugate base of peroxide ($^1HO_2^-$) producing a dioxetane (^{1}lucigenin-dioxetane) intermediate that disintegrates to a **nπ***-excited carbonyl function that relaxes to ground state by **π***-to-**n** transition with photon emission. The pK_a of $^1H_2O_2$ is 11.7. As previously considered, $^1H_2O_2$ is the sum product of two RE reductions of $^3O_2$. Consequently, lucigenin chemiluminescence is the product of reductive dioxygenation. Both lucigenin and peroxide are singlet multiplicity reactants. Spin restriction is not a problem. Alkalinity favors the formation of $^1HO_2^-$ and dioxygenation yielding a dioxetane.

Lucigenin is a heterocyclic compound with resonance and electron delocalization possibilities, and can undergo one RE reduction yielding a doublet multiplicity product (^{2}lucigenin$_{+RE}^+$). Such reduction may involve $^2O_2^-$ or some other 1RE reductant. The product radical, ^{2}lucigenin$_{+RE}^+$, can now react with $^2O_2^-$ by SOMO-SOMO overlap, that is, a doublet-doublet annihilation, producing a singlet multiplicity product, the ^{1}lucigenin-dioxetane intermediate. As depicted in **Figure 8**, the disintegration of this unstable dioxetane yields chemiluminescence [52, 58, 62, 63].

Reduction of lucigenin by 2RE, that is, by a bosonic orbital electron couple, maintains singlet multiplicity. Such a reduced ^{1}lucigenin$_{+2RE}$ can react with $^1O_2^*$, but not $^3O_2$, to produce chemiluminescence [64]. As shown in **Figure 8**, the state of lucigenin reduction determines the deoxygenating agent required. All reactions shown satisfy the spin conservation rules.

The radical product of 1RE reduction of lucigenin, ^{2}lucigenin$_{+RE}^+$, can react with the radical product of NADPH oxidase, $^2O_2^-$, resulting in intermediate dioxetane formation with breakdown to a **nπ*** electronically excited carbonyl with relaxation by light emission, and as such, lucigenin can be applied as a chemiluminigenic probe for measurement of NADPH oxidase activity [52, 58, 63]. MPO haloperoxidase activity does not yield lucigenin-luminescence.

Chicken blood phagocytes, that is, heterophil leukocytes, have oxidase activity, but are deficient in haloperoxidase. Chemical or phagocytic stimulation of these heterophil leukocytes results in lucigenin-dependent luminescence responses comparable to those observed from human neutrophils under similar test conditions and using similar stimuli [58, 65]. However, the luminol-dependent luminescence responses of MPO-deficient chicken heterophils are a hundredfold lower than those observed from MPO-rich human neutrophils. In addition, azide (N_3^-), a known inhibitor of MPO, inhibits the luminol-dependent luminescence responses of MPO-rich human neutrophil. Azide shows no inhibitory action against the luminol or the lucigenin luminescence responses of MPO-deficient chicken heterophils [66]. These chicken heterophil results plus the previously described macrophage results [57] experimentally support the position that luminol provides a very sensitive measure of MPO activity. However, the weaker luminol-luminescence measured is evidence for haloperoxidase-independent oxidase activity.

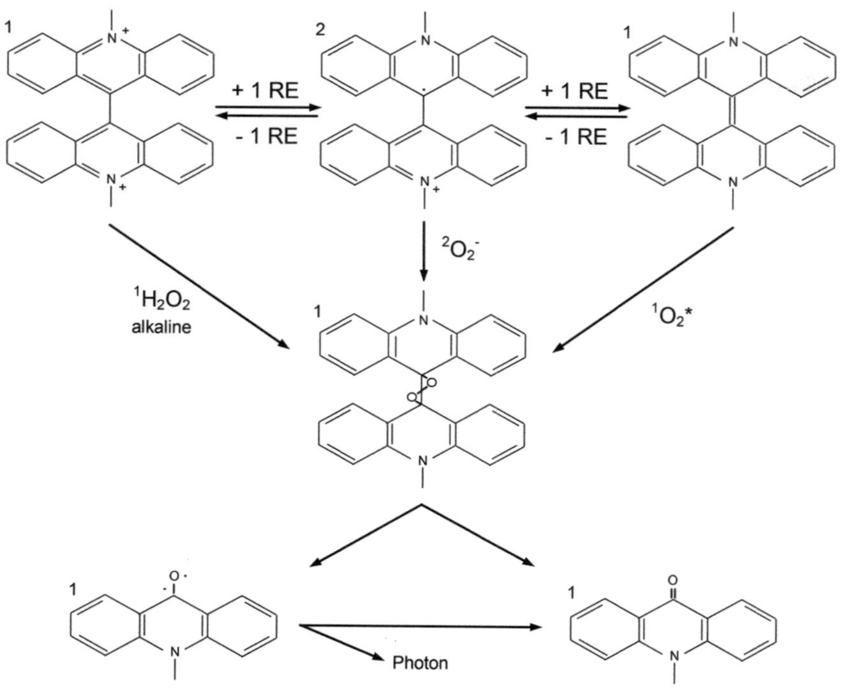

Figure 8.
Oxygenating reactions yielding lucigenin chemiluminescence. Spin multiplicity is shown by the superscript value that precedes the reactant, and 1RE indicates one reducing equivalent.

6.2 Probing oxygenation activities with cyclic hydrazides

Luminol chemiluminescence is a well-established phenomenon, but the mechanisms responsible for luminol-luminescence are diverse [67]. Luminol (5-amino-2,3-dihydrophthalazine-1,4-dione) is a nonradical, cyclic hydrazide [68]. Luminol dioxygenation is thought to involve an intermediate endoperoxide with disintegration yielding the **nπ*** electronically excited aminophthalate that relaxes by photon emission. Albrecht first described the blood-catalyzed luminol-luminescence [69]. Like lucigenin, alkalinity and $^1H_2O_2$ are required, but luminol-luminescence has an additional requirement for a catalyst, for example, blood or peroxidase. To appreciate how these CLS differ, compare, and contrast the net reactions responsible for luminol-luminescence and lucigenin-luminescence. Luminol-luminescence is a dioxygenation:

$$^1\text{luminol} + {}^3O_2 \text{—X}\rightarrow {}^1\text{aminophthalate} + {}^1N_2 + \text{Photon} \tag{14}$$

The reaction of ^{1}luminol with $^3O_2$ (Eq. (14)) is not spin allowed, but reaction with $^1O_2{}^*$ (Eq. (15)) is spin allowed producing **nπ*** electronically excited ^{1}aminophthalate* plus $^1N_2$, and ultimately, ground state ^{1}aminophthalate plus a photon.

$$^1\text{luminol} + {}^1O_2{}^* \rightarrow {}^1\text{aminophthalate} + {}^1N_2 + \text{Photon} \tag{15}$$

Lucigenin-luminescence is a reductive dioxygenation.

$$^1\text{lucigenin} + {}^1H_2O_2 \rightarrow 2\,{}^1\text{N-methylacrodone} + \text{Photon} \tag{16}$$

As per Eq. (16), lucigenin-luminescence requires the spin-allowed reactive addition of molecular oxygen plus 2RE, that is, $^1H_2O_2$. The product of this reductive dioxygenation is a dioxetane intermediate that breaks down to one ground state ^{1}N-methylacridone and one **nπ***electronically excited ^{1}N-methylacridone*. Relaxation of the ^{1}N-methylacridone* yields a photon.

Luminol dioxygenation is not reductive. The net dioxygenation incorporates molecular oxygen to produce an endoperoxide intermediate with the breakdown release of $^1N_2$ and formation of a **nπ***electronically excited aminophthalate. As indicated by Eq. (14), ^{1}luminol does not react with ground state oxygen. Spin conservation and frontier orbital overlap problems restrict such direct reaction. As illustrated in **Figure 1**, the frontier orbitals of $^3O_2$ are its two degenerates **π*** SOMOs. Hund's maximum multiplicity rule is satisfied when the electrons of each SOMO have the same spin. Each of the two **π*** orbitals of $^3O_2$ have fermionic character that restricts overlap with the bosonic frontier orbitals of luminol. By contrast, the frontier **π*** orbitals of $^1O_2{}^*$ are bosonic and include one LUMO **π*** orbital and one HOMO **π*** orbital. Overlap of the LUMO of $^1O_2{}^*$ with the HOMO of ^{1}luminol satisfies the symmetry requirements for reaction.

There are three mechanistic possibilities for ^{1}luminol reactions yielding luminescence. The fermionic (doublet multiplicity/radical) pathway requires two steps as illustrated by Eqs. (17) and (18).

$$^1\text{luminol} + {}^1H_2O_2\text{—peroxidase} \rightarrow {}^2\text{luminol}_{-1RE} + {}^1H_2O \tag{17}$$

The radical ^{2}luminol$_{-1RE}$ can participate in SOMO-SOMO reaction with superoxide ($^2O_2{}^-$) yielding singlet multiplicity electronically excited aminophthalate (^{1}aminophthalate*) that relaxes with photon emission.

$$^2\text{luminol}_{-1RE} + {}^2O_2{}^- \rightarrow {}^1\text{aminophthalate} + {}^1N_2 + \text{Photon} \tag{18}$$

The bosonic (singlet multiplicity/nonradical) pathway can occur by a single reaction as illustrated by Eq. (19),

$$^1\text{luminol} + {}^1O_2{}^* \rightarrow {}^1\text{aminophthalate}^- + {}^1N_2 + \text{Photon} \tag{19}$$

The bosonic (singlet multiplicity/nonradical) pathway can also occur by a two-step reaction as illustrated by Eqs. (20) and (21).

$$^1\text{luminol} + {}^1OCl^- \rightarrow {}^1\text{luminol}_{-2RE} + {}^1Cl^- \tag{20}$$

$$^1\text{luminol}_{-2RE} + {}^1H_2O_2 \rightarrow {}^1\text{aminophthalate} + {}^1N_2 + \text{Photon} \tag{21}$$

Although luminol is versatile with regard to reactive mechanism, dioxygenation is ultimately required for chemiluminescence. In an alkaline milieu, classical peroxidase or hemoglobin can catalyze $^1H_2O_2$-dependent luminol-luminescence. The peroxidase-catalyzed mechanism of luminol-luminescence described by Dure and Cormier illustrates the kinetics of the fermionic pathway [70]. For such reaction, a classical peroxidase is first oxidized by $^1H_2O_2$, that is, 2RE are transferred to $^1H_2O_2$ producing two ^1H_2O as described in Eq. (22).

$$\text{peroxidase} + {}^1H_2O_2 \rightarrow \text{Cpx }1_{-2RE} + 2{}^1H_2O \tag{22}$$

This 2RE oxidized peroxidase, referred to as complex 1 (Cpx 1), can now readily oxidize ^{1}luminol by removing 1RE producing ^{2}luminol$_{-1RE}$, as per Eq. (23).

$$^{1}\text{luminol} + \text{Cpx 1}_{\text{-2RE}} \rightarrow \text{Cpx 2}_{\text{-RE}} + {}^{2}\text{luminol}_{\text{-1RE}} \tag{23}$$

The reaction of complex 2 (Cpx $2_{\text{-RE}}$) with another ^{1}luminol is slow and rate limiting with regard to luminescence, but this reaction is necessary for regeneration of the starting peroxidase, as per Eq. (24).

$$^{1}\text{luminol} + \text{Cpx 2}_{\text{-RE}} \rightarrow \text{peroxidase} + {}^{2}\text{luminol}_{\text{-1RE}} \tag{24}$$

Disproportionation of the two radical ^{2}luminol$_{\text{-1RE}}$ can proceed as a spin allowed SOMO-SOMO reaction, that is, a doublet-doublet annihilation, yielding the nonradical ^{1}luminol (starting reactant) and nonradical 2RE-oxidized luminol (^{1}luminol$_{\text{-2RE}}$).

$$2\,{}^{2}\text{luminol}_{\text{-1RE}} \rightarrow {}^{1}\text{luminol} + {}^{1}\text{luminol}_{\text{-2RE}} \tag{25}$$

As per Eq. (21), the spin-allowed reaction of ^{1}luminol$_{\text{-2RE}}$ with $^{1}H_2O_2$ yields electronically excited aminophthalate (^{1}aminophthalate*) that relaxes by photon emission.

Metalloenzymes and cytochromes are suited to 1RE transfers and under proper reaction conditions can catalyze the 1RE oxidation of a ^{1}substrate producing ^{2}substrate$_{\text{-1RE}}$. The $^{1}H_2O_2$-dependent oxidation of peroxidase to Cpx $1_{\text{-2RE}}$ allows it to catalyze the initial fermionic 1RE oxidation of luminol in an alkaline milieu. Hemoglobin has peroxidase activity under alkaline conditions, thus explaining the sensitivity of luminol-luminescence for detecting the presence of blood erythrocytes by alkaline peroxide methods. Luminol-luminescence by the classical plant peroxidase-catalyzed reactions of Eqs. (22)–(25) is sensitive to pH, decreasing with increasing acidity. Acidification of the reaction milieu to a pH of about 5 ± 1 effectively eliminates classical peroxidase-catalyzed luminol luminescence. This is quantitatively demonstrated in the Michaelis-Menten enzyme kinetic analyses of luminol-luminescence for myeloperoxidase and horse radish peroxidase presented in **Table 2** [71].

Alkaline pH favors the fermionic luminol-luminescence reactions catalyzed by plant peroxidase, hemoglobin, and heavy metals. The pKa of $^{1}H_2O_2$ is 11.75. The ferricyanide-catalyzed luminol luminescence reaction is most efficient in the pH range from 10.4 to 10.8 [72]. In **Table 2**, note that no significant luminescence is observed from HRP-catalyzed luminol reaction at pH 4.9. The maximum luminescence velocity (V_{max}) values are low and standard errors (SE) are high. However, a relatively weak but significant luminescence is observed at pH 7.0, that is, Michaelis-Menten analysis of the HRP luminescence shows a low V_{max}, but an acceptable SE.

Of special note, Michaelis-Menten kinetic analysis indicates that the HRP-catalyzed luminol-luminescence velocity is first order with respect to H_2O_2 concentration, but second order with respect to luminol concentration, that is, the luminescence velocity is directly proportional to the square of the luminol concentration. These results are consistent with those reported by Dure and Cormier [70], and with the fermionic radical reactive pathway described in Eqs. (22)–(25) and Eq. (21).

Although luminol solubility becomes a problem at low pH, acidity favors the bosonic haloperoxidase luminol-luminescence catalyzed by MPO. Note that bosonic, haloperoxidase-catalyzed luminol luminescence is first order with respect to luminol, chloride, or bromide, but second order with respect to H_2O_2, that is, luminescence activity is proportional to the square of the H_2O_2 concentration.

The MPO-catalyzed luminol-luminescence kinetic finding is the opposite of those observed for HRP-catalyzed luminol-luminescence, and are consistent with the bosonic reactive pathway for luminol-luminescence via $^{1}O_2^{*}$ reaction described

	Substrate [S], variable (conc. range)	pH	Substrates, constant				Michaelis-Menten kinetics		
			H_2O_2, mM	Cl^-, mEq/L	Br^-, mEq/L	Luminol, μM	M-M equation	Km ± SE	Vmax ± SE
Haloperoxidase: Myeloperoxidase	H_2O_2 (0.01–1.4 mM)	5.0	variable	90	0	77	$v = Vmax[S]^2/(Km + [S])^2$	2.82 ± 0.05	3900 ± 1
	H_2O_2 (0.01–1.4 mM)	5.0	variable	0	4.5	77	$v = Vmax[S]^2/(Km + [S])^2$	0.58 ± 0.03	2932 ± 2
	Cl^- (0.2–7.7 mEq/L)	5.0	2.27	variable	0	45	$v = Vmax[S]/Km + [S]$	7.60 ± 2.60	1105 ± 253
	Br^- (14–882 μEq/L)	5.0	2.27	0	variable	45	$v = Vmax[S]/Km + [S]$	0.68 ± 0.05	2280 ± 96
	Luminol (0.0018–15 μM)	4.9	2.27	90	0	variable	$v = Vmax[S]/Km + [S]$	8.80 ± 0.77	1490 ± 70
	Luminol (0.0018–0.47 μM)	7.0	2.27	90	0	variable	$v = Vmax[S]/Km + [S]$	0.10 ± 0.02	3252 ± 219
Classical Peroxidase: Horse Radish Peroxidase	H_2O_2 (0.01–1.4 mM)	5.0	variable	90	0	77	$v = Vmax[S]/Km + [S]$	31.02 ± 0.05	280 ± 55
	H_2O_2 (0.01–1.4 mM)	5.0	variable	0	4.5	77	$v = Vmax[S]/Km + [S]$	17.49 ± 3.84	156 ± 34
	Cl^- (0.2–900 mEq/L)	5.0	2.27	variable	0	45	$v = Vmax[S]/Km + [S]$	0.0 ± 0.7	0 ± 0
	Br^- (14–882 μEq/L	5.0	2.27	0	variable	45	$v = Vmax[S]/Km + [S]$	6.23 ± 2.68	3 ± 0
	Luminol (0.0147–30 μM)	4.9	2.27	0	0	variable	$v = Vmax[S]^2/(Km + [S])^2$	0.0 ± 0.0	0 ± 0
	Luminol (0.0018–7.5 μM)	7.0	2.27	0	0	variable	$v = Vmax[S]^2/(Km + [S])^2$	0.90 ± 0.17	189 ± 2

Reaction milieu was 50 mM acetate buffer (pH 5.0, 4.9) or phosphate buffer (pH 7.0) in a 0.3 mL volume. The indicated conc. of Cl^- or Br^- was added in a 0.3 mL volume.

The enzymes, 78 pmol MPO and 10 pmol HRP as indicated, were added in a 0.1 mL volume. The final concentration was 78 nM for MPO and 10 nM for HRP.

The luminescence reaction was initiated by injecting the indicated concentration of H_2O_2 in a 0.3 mL volume. The final volume was 1.0 mL.
Chemiluminescence velocity (v) and Vmax are expressed as peak kilocounts of relative light units (RLU × 10–3) per sec measured during the initial 20 sec post H_2O_2 injection.

Table 2.
Michaelis-Menten enzyme kinetic analyses of classical peroxidase (horse radish peroxidase) and haloperoxidase (myeloperoxidase) activities with regard to H_2O_2, halide (Cl^- or Br^-), luminol, and pH.

in Eq. (19) or the sequential bosonic pathway described in Eqs. (20), (21). By either pathway, and consistent with the second order findings, two $^1H_2O_2$ are required for luminol dioxygenation.

Under alkaline conditions, luminol-luminescence provides high sensitivity for detection of classical peroxidase catalysts or $^1H_2O_2$, but relatively low specificity. Under acid conditions, the luminol-luminescence provides a method for specific quantification of haloperoxidase-dependent dioxygenation activity. In **Table 2**, note that Cl^- or Br^- is required for MPO-catalyzed luminol-luminescence, that the requirement is first order with respect to halide, and that the Michaelis constant (K_M) for the more electronegative Cl^- is expectedly greater that for Br^-. Haloperoxidase activity is exclusively bosonic. Reactants are all singlet multiplicity, involving HOMO-LUMO frontier orbital interaction.

Luminol was the first, and remains the most common, chemiluminigenic probe used for measurement of phagocyte oxygenation activities. Its original application was an attempt to amplify the relatively weak native luminescence signal from stimulated macrophages. Comparing the luminol-luminescence responses of neutrophils with those of macrophages illustrates that the MPO-rich neutrophils responses are several magnitudes greater than the luminol-luminescence responses from MPO-deficient macrophage [57].

Comparing MPO-rich human neutrophils with the MPO-deficient heterophile leukocytes of chickens further illustrates how chemiluminigenic probing can be used as a sensitive method for quantifying and differentiating the oxygenating activities of phagocytes [58, 65]. The luminol-dependent activities of MPO-positive human neutrophil leukocytes are a hundredfold higher than those of MPO-negative chicken heterophil leukocytes. Despite the diminution in luminol-luminescence, dioxygenation activity is still quantifiable from MPO-negative phagocytes. Such activity is not inhibited by the MPO inhibitor azide (N_3^-) [66]. In the absence of haloperoxidase, luminol-luminescence most probably reflects the type of fermionic oxidase-dependent reactions described in reactions Eqs. (17)–(18).

7. Circulating neutrophils reflect the state of inflammation

Under normal conditions, large numbers of neutrophils are produced by the hematopoietic marrow and released into the circulating blood each day, highlighting the importance of neutrophils for innate host protection against infection. To accomplish its microbicidal role, neutrophils undergo specific degranulation and mobilization of appropriate membrane receptors in response to a constellation of microbial peptides, complement activation products, cytokines, interleukins, and lipid activators. Such activities prepare neutrophils for phagocytosis, but do not directly trigger respiratory burst activity [73]. Priming actuates neutrophil locomotion and increases neutrophil recognition of and phagocytic response to opsonin-labeled microbes [56, 74, 75].

Activation of systemic inflammation in response to infection directly affects circulating blood neutrophils. The chemical signals of inflammation alter the state of neutrophil alert. As such, the state of neutrophil priming reflects the state of host immune activation [76]. Selective *in vitro* measurement of unprimed and maximally-primed circulating blood neutrophil activities by sensitive chemiluminigenic probing allows rapid multi-metric analysis using less than a half drop of anticoagulated whole blood. Analysis of such blood neutrophil luminescence metrics using classification statistical approaches, especially discriminant function analysis, allows assessment of the *in vivo* state of immune activation. The state of neutrophil priming gauges the state of host systemic inflammation [77, 78].

Acknowledgements

I gratefully acknowledge all who assisted in my education, especially my deceased mother Gladys L. Puig, my undergraduate professor Dr. Walter L. Scott Jr., my deceased mentor Dr. Richard H. Steele, and my friend and colleague Dr. Randolph M. Howes.

Conflict of interest

I am the inventor of pending and issued patents related to diagnostic applications of chemiluminescence for quantifying neutrophil function and for gauging systemic immune activation, and patents related to therapeutic applications of haloperoxidases.

Author details

Robert C. Allen
Department of Pathology, Creighton University School of Medicine, Omaha, NE, USA

*Address all correspondence to: robertallen@creighton.edu

References

[1] Northrop JH. Biochemists, biologists, and William of Occam. Annual Review of Biochemistry. 1961;**30**(1):10

[2] Allen RC, Stjernholm RL, Benerito RR, Steele RH. Functionality of electronic excitation states in human microbicidal activity. In: Chemiluminescence and Bioluminescence. Athens, GA. New York: Plenum Press; 1973. p. 498

[3] Sbarra AJ, Karnovsky ML. The biochemical basis of phagocytosis. I. Metabolic changes during the ingesting of particles by polymorphonuclear leukocytes. Journal of Biological Chemistry. 1959;**234**(4):1355-1362

[4] Allen RC, Stjernholm RL, Steele RH. Evidence for the generation of an electronic excitation state (s) in human polymorphonuclear leukocytes and its participation in bactericidal activity. Biochemical and Biophysical Research Communications. 1972;**47**(4):679-684

[5] Bazin S, Delanney A, Avice C. Le glycogène intraleucocytaire et ses variations au cours de la phagocytose. Annales de l'Institut Pasteur. 1953;**85**:774-783

[6] Stahelin H, Suter E, Karnovsky ML. Studies on the interaction between phagocytes and tubercle bacilli. I. Observations on the metabolism of Guinea pig leucocytes and the influence of phagocytosis. Journal of Experimental Medicine. 1956;**104**(1):121-136

[7] Baldridge CW, Gerard RW. The extra respiration of phagocytosis. American Journal of Physiology. 1932;**103**(1):235-236

[8] Suelter CH, Metzler DE. The oxidation of a reduced pyridine nucleotide analog by flavins. Biochimica et Biophysica Acta. 1960;**44**:23-33

[9] Michaelis L, Schwarzenbach G. The intermediate forms of oxidation-reduction of the flavins. Journal of Biological Chemistry. 1938;**123**:527-542

[10] Beinert H. Spectral characteristics of flavins at the semiquinoid oxidation level 1. Journal of the American Chemical Society. 1956;**78**(20):5323-5328

[11] Mahler HR, Cordes EH. Biological Chemistry. 2nd ed. New York: Harper and Row; 1971

[12] Massey V, Strickland S, Mayhew SG, Howell LG, Engel PC, Matthews RG, et al. The production of superoxide anion radicals in the reaction of reduced flavins and flavoproteins with molecular oxygen. Biochemical Biophysical Research Communications. 1969;**36**(6):891-897

[13] Knowles P, Gibson J, Pick F, Bray R. Electron-spin-resonance evidence for enzymic reduction of oxygen to a free radical, the superoxide ion. Biochemical Journal. 1969;**111**(1):53-58

[14] Allen RC. Oxygen-dependent microbe killing by phagocyte leukocytes: Spin conservation and reaction rate. Studies in Organic Chemistry. 1987;**33**:425-434

[15] Allen RC, Yevich SJ, Orth RW, Steele RH. The superoxide anion and singlet molecular oxygen: Their role in the microbicidal activity of the polymorphonuclear leukocyte. Biochemical and Biophysical Research Communications. 1974;**60**(3):909-917

[16] Sudbery A. Quantum Mechanics and the Particles of Nature. Cambridge: Cambridge University Press; 1986

[17] Matthews P. Quantum Chemistry of Atoms and Molecules. Cambridge: Cambridge University Press; 1986

[18] Fukui K, Yonezawa T, Shingu H. A molecular orbital theory of reactivity in aromatic hydrocarbons. Journal of Chemical Physics. 1952;**20**(4):722

[19] Allen RC. Neutrophil leukocyte: Combustive microbicidal action and chemiluminescence. Journal of Immunology Research. 2015;**15**:794072. DOI: 10.1155/2015/794072

[20] Allen RC. Molecular oxygen (O2): Reactivity and luminescence. In: Bioluminescence and Chemiluminescence: Progress & Current Applications. Cambridge UK: World Scientific; 2002. pp. 223-232

[21] Wigner E, Witmer EE. Ober die struktur der zweiatomigen molekelspektren nach der quantenmechanik. Zeitschrift für Physik. 1928;**51**:859-886

[22] Herzberg G. Molecular Spectra and Molecular Structure. Spectra of Diatomic Molecules. New York: Van Nostrand Reinhold; 1950

[23] Kasha M, Khan A. The physics, chemistry, and biology of singlet molecular oxygen. Annals of the New York Academy of Sciences. 1970;**171**:1-33

[24] Katriel J, Pauncz R. Theoretical interpretation of Hund's rule. Advances in Quantum Chemistry. 1977;**10**:143-185

[25] Allen RC. Reduced, radical, and excited state oxygen in leukocyte microbicidal activity. Frontiers of Biology. 1979;**48**:197-233

[26] Babior BM, Lambeth JD, Nauseef W. The neutrophil NADPH oxidase. Archives of Biochemistry and Biophysics. 2002;**397**(2):342-344

[27] Brandes RP, Weissmann N, Schroder K. Nox family NADPH oxidases: Molecular mechanisms of activation. Free Radical Biology and Medicine. 2014;**76**:208-226

[28] Jones RD, Hancock JT, Morice AH. NADPH oxidase: A universal oxygen sensor? Free Radical Biology and Medicine. 2000;**29**(5):416-424

[29] Skonieczna M, Hejmo T, Poterala-Hejmo A, Cieslar-Pobuda A, Buldak RJ. NADPH oxidases. Insights into selected functions and mechanisms of action in cancer and stem cells. Oxidative Medicine and Cellular Longevity. 2017;**2017**. Article ID 9420539

[30] Bielski BHJ, Allen AO. Mechanism of the disproportionation of superoxide radicals. The Journal of Physical Chemistry. 1977;**81**(11):1048-1050

[31] Behar D, Czapski G, Rabani J, Dorfman LM, Schwarz HA. Acid dissociation constant and decay kinetics of the perhydroxyl radical. The Journal of Physical Chemistry. 1970;**74**(17):3209-3213

[32] Khan AU. Singlet molecular oxygen from superoxide anion and sensitized fluorescence of organic molecules. Science. 1970;**168**(3930):476-477

[33] Dirac PAM. The Principles of Quantum Mechanics. 4th ed. Oxford: Oxford University Press; 1958

[34] Schultz J, Kaminker K. Myeloperoxidase of the leukocyte of normal human blood. I. Content and location. Archives of Biochemistry and Biophysics. 1962;**96**(3):465-467

[35] Agner K. Crystalline myeloperoxidase. Acta Chemica Scandinavica. 1958;**12**(1):89-94

[36] Bainton DF. Developmental biology of neutrophils and eosinophils. In: Gallin JI, Snyderman R, editors. Inflammation Basic Principles and Clinical Correlates. 3rd ed. Philadelphia: Lippincott Williams & Wilkins; 1999. pp. 13-34

[37] Allen RC, Stevens PR, Price TH, Chatta GS, Dale DC. In vivo effects of recombinant human granulocyte colony-stimulating factor on neutrophil oxidative functions in normal human volunteers. Journal of Infectious Diseases. 1997;**175**(5):1184-1192

[38] Allen RC. Halide dependence of the myeloperoxidase-mediated antimicrobial system of the polymorphonuclear leukocyte in the phenomenon of electronic excitation. Biochemical and Biophysical Research Communications. 1975;**63**(3):675-683

[39] Allen RC. The role of pH in the chemiluminescent response of the myeloperoxidase-halide-HOOH antimicrobial system. Biochemical and Biophysical Research Communications. 1975;**63**(3):684-691

[40] Klebanoff SJ. Myeloperoxidase-halide-hydrogen peroxide antibacterial system. Journal of Bacteriology. 1968;**95**(6):2131-2138

[41] Allen LC. Electronegativity is the average one-electron energy of the valence-shell electrons in ground-state free atoms. Journal of the American Chemical Society. 1989;**111**(25):9003-9014

[42] Pourbaix M. Atlas of Electrochemical Equilibria in Aqueous Solutions. Houston TX: National Association of Corrosion Engineers; 1974

[43] Steinbeck MJ, Khan AU, Karnovsky MJ. Intracellular singlet oxygen generation by phagocytosing neutrophils in response to particles coated with a chemical trap. Journal of Biological Chemistry. 1992;**267**(19):13425-13433

[44] Allen RC, Stephens JT Jr. Myeloperoxidase selectively binds and selectively kills microbes. Infection and Immunity. 2011;**79**(1):474-485

[45] Skovsen E, Snyder JW, Lambert JD, Ogilby PR. Lifetime and diffusion of singlet oxygen in a cell. Journal of Physical Chemistry B. 2005;**109**(18):8570-8573

[46] Redmond RW, Kochevar IE. Spatially resolved cellular responses to singlet oxygen. Photochemistry and Photobiology. 2006;**82**(5):1178-1186

[47] Allen RC, Stephens JT Jr. Reduced-oxidized difference spectral analysis and chemiluminescence-based Scatchard analysis demonstrate selective binding of myeloperoxidase to microbes. Luminescence. 2011;**26**(3):208-213

[48] Allen RC, Stephens JT Jr. Role of lactic acid bacteria-myeloperoxidase synergy in establishing and maintaining the normal flora in man. Food and Nutrition Sciences. 2013;**4**:67-72

[49] Wright DG, Meierovics AI, Foxley JM. Assessing the delivery of neutrophils to tissues in neutropenia. Blood. 1986;**67**(4):1023-1030

[50] Cauci S, Guaschino S, De Aloysio D, Driussi S, De Santo D, Penacchioni P, et al. Interrelationships of interleukin-8 with interleukin-1beta and neutrophils in vaginal fluid of healthy and bacterial vaginosis positive women. Molecular Human Reproduction. 2003;**9**(1):53-58

[51] Turro NJ, Ramamurthy V, Scaiano JC. Principles of Molecular Photochemistry. Sausalito: University Science Books; 2009

[52] Allen RC. Biochemiexcitation: Chemiluminescence and the study of biological oxygenation. In: Adam W, Cilento G, editors. Chemical and Biological Generation of Excited States. New York: Academic Press; 1982. pp. 310-344

[53] Kearns DR, Khan AU. Sensitized photooxygenation reactions and the role

of singlet oxygen. Photochemistry and Photobiology. 1969;**10**(3):193-210

[54] Allen RC, Stjernholm RL, Reed MA, Harper TB, Gupta S, Steele RH, et al. Correlation of metabolic and chemiluminescent responses of granulocytes from three female siblings with chronic granulomatous disease. Journal of Infectious Diseases. 1977;**136**(4):510-518

[55] Allen RC, Mills EL, McNitt TR, Quie PG. Role of myeloperoxidase and bacterial metabolism in chemiluminescence of granulocytes from patients with chronic granulomatous disease. Journal of Infectious Diseases. 1981;**144**(4):344-348

[56] Allen RC. Evaluation of serum opsonic capacity by quantitating the initial chemiluminescent response from phagocytizing polymorphonuclear leukocytes. Infection and Immunity. 1977;**15**(3):828-833

[57] Allen RC, Loose LD. Phagocytic activation of a luminol-dependent chemiluminescence in rabbit alveolar and peritoneal macrophages. Biochemical and Biophysical Research Communications. 1976;**69**(1):245-252

[58] Allen RC. Phagocytic leukocyte oxygenation activities and chemiluminescence: A kinetic approach to analysis. Methods in Enzymology. 1986;**133**:449-493

[59] Park BH, Fikrig SM, Smithwick EM. Infection and Bitroblue-tetrazolium reduction by neutrophils: A diagnostic aid. The Lancet. 1968;**292**(7567):532-534

[60] Ochs HD, Igo RP. The NBT slide test: A simple screening method for detecting chronic granulomatous disease and female carriers. The Journal of Pediatrics. 1973;**83**(1):77-82

[61] Gleu K, Petsch W. Die Chemiluminescenz der dimethyl-diacridyliumsalze. Angewandte Chemie. 1935;**48**(3):57-59

[62] Totter JR. The quantum yield of the chemiluminescence of dimethylbiacridinium nitrate and the mechanism of its enzymatically induced chemiluminescence. Photochemistry and Photobiology. 1964;**3**:231-241

[63] Allen RC. Lucigenin chemiluminescence: A new approach to the study of polymorphonuclear leukocyte redox activity. In: Bioluminescence and Chemiluminescence Basic Chemistry and Analytical Applications. New York: Academic Press; 1981. pp. 63-73

[64] McCapra F, Hann RA. The chemiluminescent reaction of singlet oxygen with 10, 10′-dimethyl-9, 9′-biacridylidene. Journal of the Chemical Society D: Chemical Communications. 1969;**9**:442-443

[65] Merrill GA, Bretthauer R, Wright-Hicks J, Allen RC. Oxygenation activities of chicken polymorphonuclear leukocytes investigated by selective chemiluminigenic probes. Laboratory Animal Science. 1996;**46**(5):530-538

[66] Merrill GA, Bretthauer R, Wright-Hicks J, Allen RC. Effects of inhibitors on chicken polymorphonuclear leukocyte oxygenation activity measured by use of selective chemiluminigenic substrates. Comparative Medicine. 2001;**51**(1):16-21

[67] Roswell DF, White EH. The chemiluminescence of luminol and related hydrazides. Methods in Enzymology. 1978;**57**:409-423

[68] Lind J, Merenyi G, Eriksen TE. Chemiluminescence mechanism of cyclic hydrazides such as luminol in aqueous solutions. Journal of the American Chemical Society. 1983;**105**(26):7655-7661

[69] Albrecht HO. Über die chemiluminescenz des aminophthalsäurehydrazids. Zeitschrift für Physikalische Chemie. 1928;**136U**:321-330

[70] Dure LS, Cormier MJ. Studies on the bioluminescence of Balanoglossus biminiensis extracts. Journal of Biological Chemistry. 1964;**239**:2351-2359

[71] Allen RC. Haloperoxidase Acid Optimum Chemiluminescence Assay System. USPO. Patent US005556758A1996. pp. 1-46

[72] Seitz RW. Chemiluminescence detection of enzymically generated peroxide. Methods in Enzymology. 1978;**57**:445-462

[73] Allen RC, Stevens DL. The circulating phagocyte reflects the in vivo state of immune defense. Current Opinion in Infectious Diseases. 1992;**5**(3):389-398

[74] Madonna GS, Allen RC. Shigella sonnei phase I and phase II: Susceptibility to direct serum lysis and opsonic requirements necessary for stimulation of leukocyte redox metabolism and killing. Infection and Immunity. 1981;**32**(1):153-159

[75] Allen RC, Lieberman MM. Kinetic analysis of microbe opsonification based on stimulated polymorphonuclear leukocyte oxygenation activity. Infection and Immunity. 1984;**45**(2):475-482

[76] Stevens DL, Bryant AE, Huffman J, Thompson K, Allen RC. Analysis of circulating phagocyte activity measured by whole blood luminescence: Correlations with clinical status. Journal of Infectious Diseases. 1994;**170**(6):1463-1472

[77] Taylor F, Haddad P, Kinasewitz G, Chang A, Peer G, Allen RC. Luminescence studies of the phagocyte response to endotoxin infusion into normal human subjects: Multiple discriminant analysis of luminescence response and correlation with phagocyte morphologic changes and release of elastase. Journal of Endotoxin Research. 2000;**6**(1):3-15

[78] Allen RC, Dale DC, Taylor FB. Blood phagocyte luminescence: Gauging systemic immune activation. Methods in Enzymology. 2000;**305**:591-629